NETTER'S
MOVING
ANATO*Me*

AN INTERACTIVE GUIDE TO
MUSCULOSKELETAL ANATOMY

NETTER'S MOVING ANATO*Me*

AN INTERACTIVE GUIDE TO MUSCULOSKELETAL ANATOMY

Stephanie Marango, MD, RYT
New York, New York

Carrie McCulloch, MD, RYT
New York, New York

ELSEVIER

NETTER'S MOVING ANATOME: AN INTERACTIVE GUIDE
TO MUSCULOSKELETAL ANATOMY
FIRST EDITION

ISBN: 978-0-323-56733-6

Notices

Knowledge and best practice in this field are constantly changing. As new research and experience broaden our understanding, changes in research methods, professional practices, or medical treatment may become necessary.

Practitioners and researchers must always rely on their own experience and knowledge in evaluating and using any information, methods, compounds, or experiments described herein. In using such information or methods they should be mindful of their own safety and the safety of others, including parties for whom they have a professional responsibility.

With respect to any drug or pharmaceutical products identified, readers are advised to check the most current information provided (i) on procedures featured or (ii) by the manufacturer of each product to be administered, to verify the recommended dose or formula, the method and duration of administration, and contraindications. It is the responsibility of practitioners, relying on their own experience and knowledge of their patients, to make diagnoses, to determine dosages and the best treatment for each individual patient, and to take all appropriate safety precautions.

To the fullest extent of the law, neither the Publisher nor the authors, contributors, or editors, assume any liability for any injury and/or damage to persons or property as a matter of products liability, negligence or otherwise, or from any use or operation of any methods, products, instructions, or ideas contained in the material herein.

The Publisher

Library of Congress Control Number: 2018952010

Executive Content Strategist: Elyse O'Grady
Senior Content Development Specialist: Marybeth Thiel
Publishing Services Manager: Catherine Jackson
Senior Project Manager: John Casey
Book Designer: Patrick Ferguson

Printed in Canada

9 8 7 6 5 4 3 2

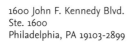

1600 John F. Kennedy Blvd.
Ste. 1600
Philadelphia, PA 19103-2899

Working together
to grow libraries in
developing countries

www.elsevier.com • www.bookaid.org

To all caretakers

Health, like happiness, is a pursuit.
May the journey inspire and move you.

ABOUT THE AUTHORS

Stephanie Marango, MD, RYT, is a physician and educator in integrative medicine. A graduate of Stanford University, Dr. Marango received her medical degree with distinction in research from the Icahn School of Medicine at Mount Sinai and trained in psychiatry at the California Pacific Medical Center. In addition to her private practice in New York, Dr. Marango is the Director of Operations for Documenting Hope, a nonprofit that studies and promotes children's health. Dr. Marango further educates about wellness at medical centers and health organizations nationwide, and her expertise is cited throughout print and broadcast media such as *Women's Health*, *Fitness*, SiriusXM, WABC radio, and WTNH TV. Dr. Marango is also a certified yoga teacher who trains movement professionals in clinical anatomy including as co-founder of the internationally renowned Functional Anatomy for Movement and Injuries (FAMI) Workshop, as well as Living AnatoME, an award-winning anatomy curriculum for medical students. She has authored a variety of works from peer-reviewed research to popular books such as *The Wisdom of Your Body* and *Your Body and The Stars*. Her work explores different perspectives on the body and how they can be employed for health and well-being.

 Carrie McCulloch, MD, RYT, is an anatomy educator and co-founder and medical director of Kinected, an integrative Pilates center in New York City specializing in injury prevention and rehabilitation. She received her medical degree with distinction in research from the Icahn School of Medicine at Mount Sinai and her bachelor's degree in journalism from the Medill School of Journalism at Northwestern University. With backgrounds in movement and medicine, she creates educational tools that connect these disciplines for both patients and professionals. She is co-founder of the Functional Anatomy for Movement and Injuries (FAMI) Workshop, an internationally renowned clinical anatomy immersion course for fitness professionals, as well as Living AnatoME, an award-winning curriculum that teaches anatomy to medical students through yoga and Pilates. In addition to her certification as a yoga teacher, Dr. McCulloch is fully certified from STOTT Pilates; her teaching and expertise, which has been featured in peer-reviewed journals and national publications such as *Vogue*, *Marie Claire*, *Fitness*, and *Pilates Style*, combine a precise understanding of the body with mindful ways of transforming health through movement.

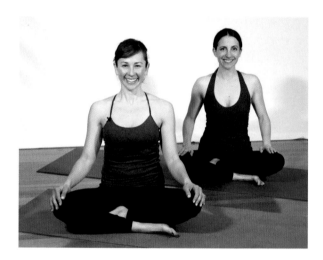

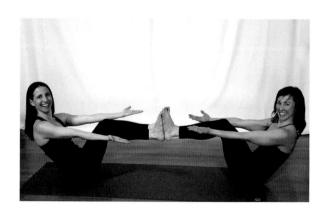

ABOUT THE ARTISTS

FRANK H. NETTER, MD

Frank H. Netter was born in New York City in 1906. He studied art at the Art Students League and the National Academy of Design before entering medical school at New York University, where he received his Doctor of Medicine degree in 1931. During his student years, Dr. Netter's notebook sketches attracted the attention of the medical faculty and other physicians, allowing him to augment his income by illustrating articles and textbooks. He continued illustrating as a sideline after establishing a surgical practice in 1933, but he ultimately opted to give up his practice in favor of a full-time commitment to art. After service in the United States Army during World War II, Dr. Netter began his long collaboration with the CIBA Pharmaceutical Company (now Novartis Pharmaceuticals). This 45-year partnership resulted in the production of the extraordinary collection of medical art so familiar to physicians and other medical professionals worldwide.

Icon Learning Systems acquired the Netter Collection in July 2000 and continued to update Dr. Netter's original paintings and to add newly commissioned paintings by artists trained in the style of Dr. Netter. In 2005, Elsevier Inc. purchased the Netter Collection and all publications from Icon Learning Systems. There are now over 50 publications featuring the art of Dr. Netter available through Elsevier Inc.

Dr. Netter's works are among the finest examples of the use of illustration in the teaching of medical concepts. The 13-book Netter Collection of Medical Illustrations, which includes the greater part of the more than 20,000 paintings created by Dr. Netter, became and remains one of the most famous medical works ever published. The Netter Atlas of Human Anatomy, first published in 1989, presents the anatomic paintings from the Netter Collection. Now translated into 16 languages, it is the anatomy atlas of choice among medical and health professions students the world over.

The Netter illustrations are appreciated not only for their aesthetic qualities, but, more importantly, for their intellectual content. As Dr. Netter wrote in 1949 "clarification of a subject is the aim and goal of illustration. No matter how beautifully painted, how delicately and subtly rendered a subject may be, it is of little value as a medical illustration if it does not serve to make clear some medical point." Dr. Netter's planning, conception, point of view, and approach are what inform his paintings and what make them so intellectually valuable.

Frank H. Netter, MD, physician and artist, died in 1991.

Learn more about the physician-artist whose work has inspired the Netter Reference collection: https://www.netterimages.com/artist-frank-h-netter.html

CARLOS MACHADO, MD

Carlos Machado was chosen by Novartis to be Dr. Netter's successor. He continues to be the main artist who contributes to the Netter collection of medical illustrations.

Self-taught in medical illustration, cardiologist Carlos Machado has contributed meticulous updates to some of Dr. Netter's original plates and has created many paintings of his own in the style of Netter as an extension of the Netter collection. Dr. Machado's photorealistic expertise and his keen insight into the physician/patient relationship inform his vivid and unforgettable visual style. His dedication to researching each topic and subject he paints places him among the premier medical illustrators at work today.

Learn more about his background and see more of his art at: https://www.netterimages.com/artist-carlos-a-g-machado.html

FOREWORD

Everyone has a body, so everyone should have an interest in their own anatomy. However, most traditional anatomy textbooks are opened with trepidation (even by those learning the medical profession). As encyclopedic listings of anatomical structures, these texts can be overwhelming. For sure, their authors have worked diligently to ensure they have listed every detail, fact-checked every fact, and even related it to common injuries or diseases. However, reading traditional textbooks can sometimes leave you with much to be desired, and more often than not, can summon slumber. As someone who has made a career of teaching anatomy, I know all too well that textbooks are not riveting reading material. Collections of facts and static images fall short in creativity, humor, passion, and relevance and thus fail "to bring it to life" for the student. That's exactly where *Netter's Moving AnatoME* differs from all other anatomy textbooks.

The authors, Stephanie Marango and Carrie McCulloch, take you on a kinesthetic journey in *Netter's Moving AnatoME.* They bring anatomy teaching to a new realm: experiential education, focused on appreciating musculoskeletal anatomy from the perspective of one's own body. The authors incorporate movement as a tool for understanding musculoskeletal anatomy. This book is aptly titled as it emphasizes the "ME" in Anatomy. In other words, the focus is on you — the person reading this book — and your personal anatomy.

As a professional educator myself, being both a medical school professor and an international television presenter for nature documentaries, I know the value of instilling creativity and relatable analogies into my teaching to engage my audience. Over the decades of my teaching, I have found that there are many ways to make the material interesting, engaging, and relatable to everyone. For example, in explaining why the ulna has an olecranon process, I may refer to a see-saw to illustrate the principles of a lever. I also demonstrate how a cat rests its arms with angled elbows, sitting like a sphinx, because unlike humans a cat cannot straighten its elbow to 180 degrees and nest the olecranon process into the humerus. Other times, to bring anatomy to life, I may incorporate drawing, even for the novice artist.

Of all of the methods I have used, the one that has garnered the most success is the incorporation of an interactive demonstration using volunteers. Movement brings 2-D structures to life, and such 3-D physicality makes the material exciting, relatable, and memorable. Think back to your childhood for a moment. Did you do hand motions along with songs to remember the body parts (e.g., "Head, shoulders, knees and toes, knees and toes…" or "The head bone's connected to the neck bone…")? If you still remember them today, then it was a successful learning session! Most adults still enjoy getting in touch with their inner child and crave a chance to learn while playing. That is what makes this book so much fun! You are no longer a mere passive learner, but instead get a chance to play along as an active participant. In other words, active learning (through doing physical activities) is actively encouraged. You will become that demo volunteer, that dancing child, and that eager student feeding the mind while embracing physicality.

This book is a culmination of the authors' skills in physicality — in teaching body movements, combined with their medical knowledge of the body (anatomy, physiology, pathology, orthopedics, etc.). Both authors are movement instructors (yoga and Pilates), and both are also physicians. It's a perfect marriage of movement and medicine, woven into a creative new textbook. As you learn anatomy from this book, you will gain a unique appreciation of your own body's physical capabilities. Hopefully, this knowledge and awareness will inspire you to promote healthy exercises that achieve and maintain wellness not only in yourself, but also within your larger community including patients and clients.

Joy S. Reidenberg, PhD
Professor of Anatomy
Center for Anatomy and Functional Morphology
Icahn School of Medicine at Mount Sinai
New York, New York

PREFACE

It's difficult to define "health." A healthy state doesn't necessarily possess the objective measures that a disease state does—like abnormal lab values, findings on imaging, etc. And while we can quantify a nondiseased state with "normal" lab values and lack of pathology, at the end of the day, health is a subjective sense that is ultimately gauged by the individual.

Do you feel healthy? What do you need to feel healthy (e.g., certain foods, favorite physical activities, amount of sleep, time spent in hobbies)? What obstacles exist between you and a healthy lifestyle? While seemingly simple questions, not everyone knows their own personal answers. But, as future health professionals, you should—for the sake of your own health, as well as the health of your patients.

And there's no better time than now. It's easy to think that time will avail itself to you in the future, like in the fourth year of medical school, or the last year of residency or fellowship or, finally, once you're an attending. But in our experience, that's not how life happens. If you don't intentionally prioritize exercise, meditation, reading, sleep—your self-care—you will fill your time with everything else instead.

Self-care is a practice. As with a muscle, the more you engage with it, the stronger it becomes. Which is why even 2 minutes of practicing **Yoga Plank Pose** every day will—3 months later—lead to a stronger core (and likely more time spent exercising it). In contrast, waiting until you find that coveted 1 hour to get to the gym will result—3 months later—in continued waiting.

So start now. Whatever your self-care practice is, use this book to enhance it, even in 2-minute intervals. Do the exercises as you read, instead of waiting until a "better" time presents itself. Allow the material to inspire you to spend more time understanding and moving the body you inhabit, engaging in regular and intentional physical activity. That's why we wrote this book—to help you be the healthiest version of you.

Your body is an amazing substrate and the only one you have. Listen to it, learn from it…it's yours for a lifetime.

Yours in health,
Drs. Marango & McCulloch

ACKNOWLEDGMENTS

We have written a book about how the parts of the body function together, as an interconnected whole. We, likewise, see the people in our lives—teachers, students, friends, colleagues, family, and more—as working together to help the book coalesce. To these individuals, we extend a heartfelt appreciation—you know who you are. To the handful of individuals who played a more direct role, we offer direct gratitude: Elyse O'Grady at Elsevier for her foresight and faith in our project; Marybeth Thiel, our editor (along with her team), for her diligence and dedication working with us; Drs. Jeffrey Laitman and Joy Reidenberg for inspiring us with anatomy in medical school; to our parents for sending us to medical school, in the first place; and, Jotin Marango and Matt McCulloch for foundational support, patience, advice (solicited and unsolicited), and love.

CONTENTS

VIDEO CONTENTS

1

Introduction to Moving AnatoME

WHY WE WROTE THIS BOOK

When we entered medical school, we both had experience as "movers": Carrie was a Pilates instructor and Stephanie a yoga teacher. With our backgrounds in movement, we were excited to learn about musculoskeletal anatomy, whether by taking part in a gross anatomy lab, poring over our atlases, or joining a study group. Although these educational resources offered vast amounts of information, we soon realized that something was missing: We wanted to learn about anatomy in relationship to our own bodies. Simultaneously, we were craving more movement for our bodies because we had less and less time for exercise and more and more strain from studying. Out of this quandary was born the idea of using yoga and Pilates to study the body. We have subsequently spent years merging the fields of movement and medicine in our personal and professional lives, creating **Moving AnatoME** along the way. We have written this book as a comprehensive learning tool for doing the same in your own life.

We have found that students appreciate the approach of Moving AnatoME because it addresses three objectives at once: anatomy comprehension, physical awareness, and well-being. Both yoga and Pilates rely upon knowledge of functional anatomy and a mind-body connection; thus, incorporating the two practices into anatomy learning not only deepens a student's comprehension of *the* human body but also enhances an awareness of *her* or *his* human body. For instance, knowing that the long head of the biceps femoris extends the hip joint is not just a fact to memorize; it is also a physical reality that can be experienced and can serve as a guide for selecting exercises to strengthen the posterior thigh.

Another reason that the Moving AnatoME approach is effective is that it incorporates students' different learning paradigms and preferences. It is a multimodal teaching tool that integrates written material with a lecture format, visual demonstrations, and movement basics. It therefore encompasses all types of learners, whether they prefer visual, auditory, written, or kinesthetic methods by nature.

Moving AnatoME also addresses self-care within health education at a time when physician and nursing burnout rates are higher than ever. Burnout may begin with habits set in motion when one is a student. Although the rigors of school encourage the mastery of material, they also normalize unhealthy habits, such as not getting enough sleep, not eating balanced meals with adequate nutrition, and not exercising regularly or having enough leisure time. As unhealthy habits turn into a lifestyle, they can become a permanent way of functioning for many healthcare providers.

To stop these patterns, we urge students to hold themselves to the same standards that they would use to assess the lifestyles of their patients. Your health—as well as the health of your fellow students and teachers—is important. Because it's *your* health. And beyond that, your health has a ripple effect on your friends, family, and patients, as well. Both common sense and studies show that physicians who personally know how to eat and exercise well are better able to professionally parlay that information to others. Students should therefore be

1

encouraged to apply their ever-increasing knowledge about anatomy, health, and nutrition to themselves as part of their studies.

Regardless of your position as student, teacher, doctor, patient—or anyone else—at the end of the day, your health is ultimately your responsibility. And so it's best to practice healthy habits now because new patterns become harder to adopt—and old patterns harder to change—over time. This book provides one way to form healthy habits of movement as you proceed with your current studies. We, the authors, have been where you are, and we understand that convenience is key, not only as you follow your study schedule but also as you form patterns in general. So join the movement now (pun intended) and help healthcare by taking care of the caretaker.

WHAT'S IN THIS BOOK

This book provides the health professional with an experiential way to learn musculoskeletal anatomy and kinesiology. Its organization is movement based, allowing you to explore each region joint by joint. For each joint, we have included yoga and Pilates exercises, so you can apply what you are learning about the anatomy of each region to your own body.

There are print and online formats of this book. The print version includes written instructions and photographs of exercises, and the online version contains a video of each exercise. We hope you will find them helpful, restorative, and fun. Each format can be used as a stand-alone reference or in conjunction with the others.

The book is divided into three main parts:

Part 1: Introduction

Part 1, Introduction, has three chapters. The first introduces the subject of Moving AnatoME and describes the contents of this book. The second presents background material on yoga and Pilates. The third is a primer on movement, which explains anatomical terminology and the overarching principles of anatomy and biomechanics that govern *every* body. For anyone studying anatomy, whether a newcomer to it or a medical "veteran" returning for a review, a strong foundation is essential so that learning can take place efficiently and smoothly. Once a student understands how anatomical terms have been derived, the process of learning anatomy is transformed from rote memorization to educated reasoning. The

overarching concepts of biomechanics and kinesiology are also explained to lay the groundwork for the specific joint mechanics that are presented in Parts 2, 3, and 4. Although each joint is one piece of the body's "puzzle," there are general principles that indicate how all the pieces fit together.

Part 2: Your Axial Skeleton: Head, Neck, and Back; Part 3: Your Appendicular Skeleton: Upper Extremity; and Part 4: Your Appendicular Skeleton: Lower Extremity

In Parts 2, 3, and 4, the principles introduced in Part 1 are applied to the human body's *two* skeletons: axial and appendicular (together, they form the single skeleton with which you are familiar). The axial skeleton is, in evolutionary terms, the older skeleton and includes the skull, vertebral column, and rib cage. The appendicular skeleton, which developed millenia later, includes the pectoral girdle and upper extremities, as well as the pelvic girdle and lower extremities. There are many lenses through which one can view and study these skeletons; the lens we have chosen is movement. For each region, therefore, we have provided a brief overview to orient the reader anatomically. In Part 2, Your Axial Skeleton: Head, Neck, and Back, there are chapters on the head and the neck and back. In Part 3, Your Appendicular Skeleton: Upper Extremity, there are chapters on the shoulder, elbow, wrist, and hand. In Part 4, Your Appendicular Skeleton: Lower Extremity, there are chapters on the hip, knee, ankle, and foot. Each chapter "dissects" the body one joint at a time, delving into the structure, function, and movements of each. Here, we pare down volumes of anatomical information to illuminate the "nuts and bolts" needed to understand a joint's architecture. Although this text is not meant to be a comprehensive kinesiology book, we include biomechanical concepts so that you can see how each individual part not only functions but also how it interconnects with joints in other regions. To set things in motion (literally), each chapter details the biomechanics of the movements permitted at each joint, as well as lists the primary muscular actors and their innervations. Of note, you will see that slightly different muscular actors are discussed in different anatomical texts; we chose ours based on an integration of anatomical, orthopedic, and kinesiologic principles.

At the end of each movement summary, we highlight yoga and Pilates exercises that bring the anatomy of each joint to life, while also providing you with exercises to keep your body limber. We chose these two movement modalities—of many available—for a variety of reasons, including our expertise as teachers of them, their usefulness in demonstrating anatomy, and their value as adjuncts to mainstream healthcare (in addition to their innate value as health disciplines). Also, because yoga and Pilates are two of the most popular forms of exercise today, you may have already practiced them or can easily find classes for them if you want to begin. The featured exercises can be performed by persons at all levels of expertise, with modifications according to the needs of your particular body. The print copy of this book includes images of, as well as detailed instructions for, each exercise. You can also log onto the virtual platform to watch a video of each exercise.

Part 5: Your Body as Medicine

In Parts 1 to 4, we employed movement and physical awareness to learn anatomy. In Part 5, we transform these educational tools into self-care tools that can impact your life off the mat and outside of the classroom (ie, they are the "how" of self-care). It is one thing to know about healthy habits but another thing to practice them, let alone parlay them effectively to others.

This part's practical application focuses on posture and mindfulness. Although not covered extensively in healthcare studies, these topics can provide a good foundation for good health. They also are great starting points for practicing what you preach about movement, as well as essential touchpoints that you can return to at any time as you move along your path of self-care. Understanding how to stand efficiently (posture section) and breathe deeply (mindfulness section), for example, may not only help combat common occupational hazards but may also positively affect your patient population. For instance, engaging in the **Yoga and Pilates Flow** (see Video 18-4) can help you assume a proper stance and/or reengage your focus in the present. The tips and tools herein are ones you can apply, as needed, in your studies and throughout your life.

Practicing What We Preach and Providing a Clinical Focus

A primary goal of the book is to give you information that is as practical as possible. To this end, we have interwoven boxes titled *Practice What You Preach* and *Clinical Focus* throughout the text. The Practice What

You Preach boxes give tips on using anatomical concepts to improve your own health and function, for example, by learning how to counteract "white coat kyphosis." The Clinical Focus boxes provide basic information on dysfunction and highlight common musculoskeletal injuries and their underlying causes, as well as prognosis and implications for exercise.

HOW TO USE THIS BOOK

This book is geared to students of the human body, including medical and allied health professionals, movement and fitness professionals, physical therapists, manual therapists, and others. This book is not intended to be everything to everyone, however. Many great anatomy texts exist, and each serves its own purpose.

Our book intends to make anatomy practical. Relevant. Functional. As it is every day for your body. For that reason, we have not included the name of every single ligament or bony landmark. Our goal is not to provide a litany of facts; they already can be found in many books and online sources. Rather, we focus on applications that will get you up and using your anatomy, so that you can bring to life the information you find in this book and others.

We therefore encourage common sense and caution when using the book. The recommended exercises are intended for a broad audience, whose fitness levels vary. We may state a rule, but your body (or someone else's) may be the exception. So please modify each exercise to fit the needs of your body (eg, decreasing the depth of a lunge, using supportive cushions or blocks), and do so with diligence and self-awareness. Positioning yourself in the proper alignment while exercising is also important, as is working within a pain-free, comfortable range of motion. Ultimately, you are the expert who knows your body best.

Using this book will further help you understand your body and how it works. Although you can read it from cover to cover, we recommend that you read it as an adjunct. You likely already have at least one large anatomy atlas, such as the *Atlas of Human Anatomy,* and *Netter's Clinical Anatomy.* We hope that as you read in your atlas about the bones, muscles, and other structures of the hip, you will also turn to our book to learn *how* these structures work (ie, joint mechanics) and do the exercises to feel the structures at work in your own body. Likewise, after doing squats at the gym and wondering which structures you have been using, you can flip back to the hip chapter to refresh your understanding of the mechanics of thigh flexion and extension. We have found that anatomical material is easier to bone up on (pun intended) when you use investigation, repetition, and application.

We sincerely hope that you enjoy using this book as much as we enjoyed writing it, and that you learn as much from referring to it as we did from compiling it. The movement and medicine worlds have existed side by side for some time, and now, as a new age unfolds, there is an opportunity to bridge the gap between the two. We are honored to be part of creating this bridge and privileged to have you join us in crossing it.

Overview of Yoga and Pilates

Yoga and Pilates are two of the most popular movement modalities today. They engage tens of millions of practitioners and teachers, constituting a sector of the fitness industry that is growing "faster than average," according to the Bureau of Labor Statistics. While the practices share certain similarities, they come from different origins. Although yoga is relatively new to our society, it has been practiced for centuries in other parts of the world. The earliest records (Vedas) of its practice date to about 5000 BCE in India. Pilates, in contrast, originated in Europe during the early 20th century.

YOGA

In Sanskrit, the word *yoga* means "to yoke," or to bring together. What yoga unites are your individual and spiritual selves; it provides a body-mind-spirit balance that enables you to live a happy, healthy, and harmonious life. It is a philosophy but it also entails a practice, which may be followed through six different systems of study: Raja (path of meditation), Karma (path of service), Bhakti (path of devotion), Jnana (path of knowledge), Tantra (path of ritual), and Hatha (path of physical purification). Each path represents a different way of achieving the same goal of union. It is important to note, however, that adherence to one of these paths does not preclude any of the others; many times, the paths naturally intersect, for example, when you regularly attend yoga classes to practice poses (Hatha path), volunteer at a local shelter (Karma path), and read yoga philosophy (Jnana path).

Hatha yoga is currently the most popular path in the West. It prescribes a practice of asanas, or poses, such as the popular **Yoga Downward-Facing Dog** (see Video 11.2) and **Yoga Tree Pose** (see Video 13.1) described in this book. These asanas are typically performed in

sequence under the tutelage of a teacher in a yoga studio: Ashtanga (power yoga), bikram (hot yoga), and vinyasa (flow yoga) are all examples of modern-day manifestations of Hatha yoga.

PILATES

The Pilates method developed more recently. It was created by a man named Joseph Pilates just under a century ago. Born in Germany in 1883, Pilates suffered from asthma and other childhood ailments. He was motivated to study disciplines such as yoga, Zen meditation, and martial arts to restore his health; as he grow older he grew stronger, well enough to become a skier, gymnast, and boxer. Overall, his experiences reaffirmed his belief in the classic Greek ideal of a (wo)man balanced in body, mind, and spirit, and, accordingly, he began to develop his approach to body conditioning.

While living in England during World War I, Pilates put his knowledge into practice. Placed in a British internment camp, he began training fellow internees and subsequently developed a system of exercises that focused on principles such as core strength, breath, and proper posture. These original exercises, some of which we know today as the **Pilates Swimming** (Video 13.3) and **Pilates Spine Twist** (Video 6.4) exercises, were performed on a mat. A few years later, while working in the infirmary of another internment camp, he developed exercises and ideas for specialized equipment such as the Pilates reformer. These ideas arose from creative approaches to moving bed-bound patients, for example, by rigging the springs from cots to provide non–weight-bearing forms of resistance training.

When Pilates immigrated to the United States in 1926, he and his wife, Clara, brought his system into a studio

5

that he opened in New York City. The studio shared an address with the New York City Ballet, and the Pilates technique became popular with dancers such as Martha Graham and George Balanchine. Pilates originally called his technique Contrology; only later did it become known by his surname, and it did not enter the mainstream until years after Pilates' death.

VALUE OF YOGA AND PILATES

It wasn't until the 1970s and 1980s that the media began to widely cover yoga and Pilates, as part of an increasing interest in fitness. The public took note, and the movement disciplines entered the mainstream. Not only can they now be found in fitness facilities worldwide, but they have also become training adjuncts for elite athletes, corporate wellness tools for productive employees, and complementary alternatives to patients undergoing medical treatment.

Although the two disciplines are different, people tend to come to yoga and Pilates for similar reasons: to maintain health and wellness, to receive therapy for pain and/or injury, and to prevent injury. Practicing either discipline safely and effectively requires one to gain an understanding of and respect for functional anatomy. This understanding develops as one practices each method over time. The disciplines bring anatomy to life because they offer ample opportunities to translate anatomical fact into physical awareness and to parlay academic knowledge into daily experience. As an added bonus for students living with demanding physical or mental challenges, such as an intensive course of advanced academic study, both disciplines promote a holistic approach to well-being and provide practical tools for patients and caregivers alike.

3

A Primer on Movement

INTRODUCTION TO ANATOMICAL TERMINOLOGY

Akin to a foreign language, anatomical terminology is a complex lexicon with many unfamiliar nouns, verbs, and adjectives. It was first developed in ancient Greece and Rome by physician scientists such as Hippocrates, Galen, and later Vesalius, who explored the human body and compiled a collection of works that set the standard for anatomical studies today. Over time, the official language of anatomical nomenclature became established as Latin. The terminology has most recently been codified as the *Terminologia Anatomica,* which contains approximately 7500 terms. These terms are accepted internationally as the standard anatomical nomenclature by professionals in many fields, including the health sciences. Anatomical terminology is important to learn because it allows consistent communication across fields and cultures; for example, it allows an internist in India to communicate with a Pilates professional in Pennsylvania.

ANATOMICAL POSITION

For anatomical purposes, it is traditional to view the body in classic anatomical position (Fig. 3.1). This view provides a basic reference for describing the regions and structures of the body. The body is in anatomical position when it is standing upright with
- feet pointing forward;
- arms by the sides with the palms of the hands facing forward and fingers extended; and
- head front and center, with a neutral facial expression.

ANATOMICAL DIRECTIONS

The body is a three-dimensional entity that moves in space. Describing the relationship of one body part to

another can therefore be challenging. For instance, it may be difficult to discuss the **Yoga Wide-Legged Forward Bend** (see Video 11.1), in which the head is spatially in front of the legs but anatomically superior to them. Communication becomes easier if the standard anatomical position is used as a reference point and proper anatomical terminology is applied to describe the location of body structures. The terminology can be used for any position into which a body can twist (Fig. 3.2). The terms for the various directions of the body are

- **Superior (cranial):** above, or closer to the head (eg, the head is superior to the neck).
- **Inferior (caudal):** below, or closer to the feet (eg, the elbow is inferior to the shoulder).
- **Anterior (ventral):** closer to the front surface of the structure or body (eg, the tip of the nose is anterior to the rest of the face).
- **Posterior (dorsal):** closer to the back surface of the structure or body (eg, the hamstrings are posterior to the quadriceps).
- **Medial:** closer to the midline of the body (eg, the clavicle is medial to the humerus).
- **Lateral:** farther away from the midline of the body (eg, the humerus is lateral to the clavicle).
- **Proximal:** closer to the trunk, the origin of a muscle, or the attachment point of a limb to the body (eg, palpate the proximal tibia, just below the knee).
- **Distal:** farther from the trunk, the origin of a muscle, or the attachment point of a limb to the body (eg, palpate the distal tibia, just above the ankle).
- **Superficial:** closer to the surface of the structure or body (eg, the rectus abdominis muscle is the most superficial layer of the abdominal wall muscles).
- **Deep:** farther from the surface of the structure or body (eg, the transversus abdominis lies deep to the rectus abdominis and oblique muscles).

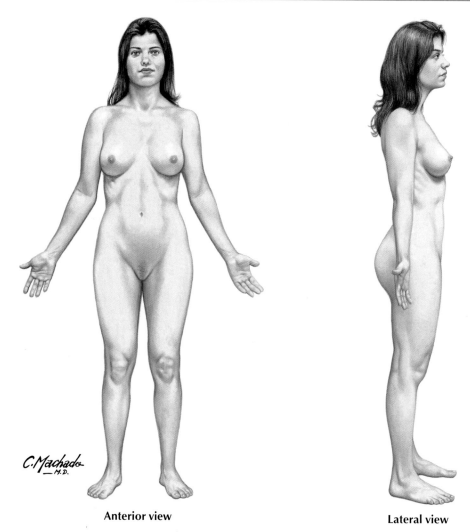

Anterior view   Lateral view

Fig. 3.1 Anatomical position of the body.

- **Palmar:** of, or referring to, the anterior surface of the hand (eg, in a push-up position, the palmar surfaces of the hands contact the floor).
- **Plantar:** of, or referring to, the inferior surface of the foot, otherwise known as the sole (eg, the plantar aspect of the foot contacts the ground when standing).

ANATOMICAL MOTION

Planes and Movements

When studying anatomy, you view the body from many different angles. Those angles are determined by the plane from which you view them. Three major planes pass through a body in anatomical position: the sagittal (median), coronal (frontal), and transverse (horizontal) planes (see Fig. 3.2). These planes are imaginary, and they "cut" through the body at any location. Medical professionals visualize the body along these planes. For example, an x-ray of the shoulder can be taken in the coronal plane (Fig. 3.3). An image produced by magnetic resonance imaging (an MRI scan) can also capture the same body part in the transverse plane. To view the shoulder sagittally, an anatomist might dissect it along the length of the humerus.

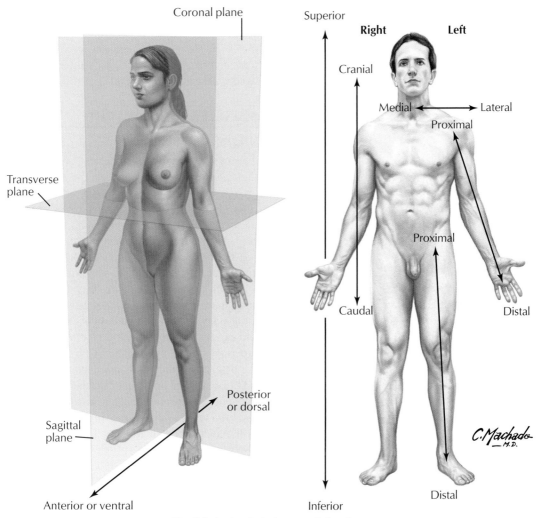

Fig. 3.2 Anatomical planes and directions.

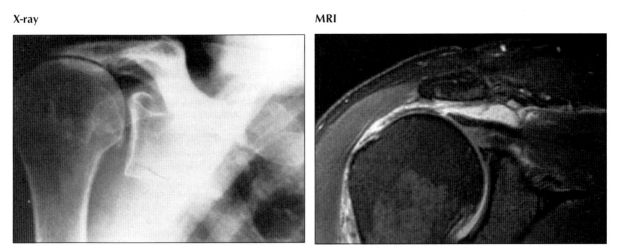

Fig. 3.3 Coronal plane: X-ray and MRI of a torn rotator cuff.

Knowledge of anatomical planes is essential for understanding how the body moves. Every movement, from flexion of the knee to supination of the forearm, occurs in some combination of the body's three cardinal planes (sagittal, coronal, and/or transverse) or in a derivation of them (eg, the near sagittal plane, which refers to a sagittal plane on a slight angle).

Axes of Rotation

Whereas planes help describe the gross movements of a limb or body part, axes of rotation help describe the kinematics happening at the joint. An axis of rotation is a specific (but imaginary) reference line about which a joint revolves. The axis of rotation is thereby perpendicular to the plane of motion. For example, the shoulder joint has three axes running through it: one longitudinal, one medial-lateral, and one anterior-posterior. During shoulder flexion, the humerus rotates around the joint's medial-lateral axis, thereby moving the arm superiorly in the sagittal plane. Abduction and adduction occur about the joint's anterior-posterior axis (moving the shoulder in the coronal plane), and internal and external rotations occur about the joint's longitudinal axis (moving the shoulder in the transverse plane).

Kinetic Chain

Another common way to describe the biomechanics of a joint involves the concept of a kinetic chain. A complex topic, kinetic chain theory acknowledges the interrelationship of joints involved in a movement; it likens them to links in a chain that can produce either open or closed motions. Though shades of gray exist between these two categories, they are generally defined as follows:

- **Open-chain motions** are those in which the distal bone of a joint moves while the proximal bone remains stable (eg, knee extension that occurs when the femur is relatively fixed and the tibia rotates around it [tibial-on-femoral extension], seen in extending the leg to kick a soccer ball).
- **Closed-chain motions** are movements in which the proximal bone of a joint moves while the distal bone remains stationary (eg, knee extension that occurs when the tibia remains relatively fixed and the femur rotates around it [femoral-on-tibial extension], seen when extending the leg to rise from a seated position).

Both types of movement occur throughout the body, but with unequal distribution. The upper extremities mainly employ open-chain, distal-on-proximal mechanics to bring objects from the environment closer to the body; the lower extremities regularly perform closed-chain movements because the distal segment (foot) is often fixed on the ground.

MUSCLES AND MOTION

Origins and Insertions

A muscle moves a bone by acting across a joint. Most muscles cross only one joint and therefore have an effect on only that joint; for instance, the brachialis crosses the elbow joint and acts on it to flex the forearm. A few muscles, including the biceps brachii, rectus femoris, and gastrocnemius, cross two joints and therefore affect both (eg, the rectus femoris flexes the hip and extends the knee [but usually not at the same time]).

To affect a joint, a muscle must be attached at sites both proximal and distal to the joint. These attachments are also known as insertion points or the point of origin and point of insertion. As a rule of thumb, the more proximal muscle attachment is typically referred to as the origin and the more distal point as the insertion. Additionally, the origin tends to be the attachment site that remains stable during a movement, whereas the insertion tends to do the moving. Take, for example, the vasti muscles of the quadriceps: To extend the knee during a soccer-ball kick, these muscles contract to move their insertion point (the tibia) while their origin (the femur) remains relatively stationary.

Sometimes, though, this rule of thumb does not apply, and the origin moves while the insertion remains stable. Take another look at the role of the vasti muscles in knee extension, this time focusing on the movement as a person stands up from a seated position: In this case, the insertion of the vasti muscles (the tibia) remains relatively stationary while the origin (the femur) moves.

To further convolute matters, both the origin and insertion of a muscle might move during a contraction, as demonstrated by the rectus abdominis during a sit-up. During this action, the rectus abdominis moves both its origin (on the rib cage) and its insertion (on the pelvis) to flex the spine and bring these points closer together.

Muscles as Movers

How many muscles does it take to flex the knee? Obviously, knee flexors such as the hamstrings are involved. But just as the hamstrings must contract in order to flex the knee, so must the quadriceps muscles relax. And then there is the matter of the popliteus muscle, which assists in "unlocking" the knee from its extended position. As you can see, it takes more than one muscle to move a body part. The following terms describe the different roles in the process:

- **Agonist (a.k.a. primary mover):** The main muscle or muscle group directly responsible for a specific movement. For example, the triceps brachii muscle is the primary extensor of the elbow.
- **Antagonist:** The muscle or muscle group that has the opposite action of a particular agonist; it must relax in order for the agonist to perform its function. For example, the biceps brachii must relax and elongate for the triceps brachii to contract.
- **Synergist:** A muscle or muscle group that facilitates the action of the agonist. For example, when the triceps contracts to extend the forearm, the anconeus muscle acts as a synergist by contracting simultaneously to facilitate a more effective extension.

Types of Muscle Contractions

A muscle contracts upon nerve stimulation. But do not confuse contraction with shortening. By definition, a muscular contraction is an activation of muscle fibers. This activation *may* result in a shortening (eg, the triceps brachii shortens when you are extending your elbows during a push-up), but it also may result in a lengthening (eg, the triceps brachii lengthens when you are slowly lowering down during a push-up) or a static increase in the muscle's tension (eg, the tension of the triceps brachii increases when you are pushing against a wall). If the contraction causes any change in length of the muscle fibers, it is considered isotonic; if no change in size occurs, the contraction is isometric.

- **Isotonic** (Greek *iso*, "equal"; *tone*, "tension"): An isotonic contraction is when a muscle maintains the same level of tension as it changes in length. Isotonic contractions are categorized according to the change in length that occurs:

- **Concentric:** Concentric contractions bring a muscle's attachments closer together, thereby shortening the muscle and moving the related joint. To kinesthetically understand this concept, bend your right elbow. To do this, you concentrically contracted your elbow flexors, such as the brachialis muscle, bringing its attachments above and below the elbow closer together.
- **Eccentric:** Eccentric contractions create distance between a muscle's attachments, thereby lengthening the muscle and moving the related joint. Beginning with your elbow bent, slowly straighten it as if moving against resistance. Notice how by lowering your forearm in a controlled fashion, you are still contracting your elbow flexors; this eccentric muscular contraction counters the effects of gravity, which, if left unchecked, would cause your forearm to fall faster and more haphazardly toward the ground.
- **Isometric** (Greek *iso*, "equal"; *meter*, "measure, length"): An isometric contraction occurs when a muscle increases its tension without changing its length. Movement does not ensue, because the joint does not move. Think about placing both hands on the side of a piano and, with elbows bent, pushing against the piano with all your might. The piano will not move, and neither will your elbows, yet you will surely feel the muscular activation involved with this isometric contraction. You isometrically contract on a daily basis without thinking twice about it. Consider the position of your head, for example; if your posterior neck extensors were not constantly working to maintain your head upright, the center of gravity of the skull would continually pull your head forward and you would spend your days walking around with forward flexion of the head and neck, eyes toward the ground.

4

Regional Overview of Axial Skeleton

There are about 206 bones in the human body (we say *about* because many small and variable bones, such as some sesamoids, a cervical rib, or an accessory navicular bone, are not included in the count). Together, all of these bones form not one, but two, skeletons. What is commonly considered to be *the* human skeleton is, in fact, a combination of two skeletons: the ancient axial skeleton, composed of the skull, ribs, and vertebral column, and the evolutionarily newer appendicular skeleton, which includes all of the bones of the upper and lower extremities. The axial skeleton forms the vertical axis of your body; it moves on its own and also enables movements of other bones, such as those of the upper and lower extremities. Its central structure is the vertebral column, or spine. (You actually have several other spines in your body, not only the one in your back; for example, the spine of the scapula and the ischial spine of the pelvis.) *Spina* is Latin for "thorn," and early anatomists adopted this term to describe the "thorny" protrusions they found throughout the body. Run your hand down the middle of your back to tangibly appreciate the derivation of this term.

Along with the vertebral column, the skull and rib cage work together to create a unified framework that supports and protects your internal organs, from the brain in your skull and spinal cord in your vertebral column, to the heart and lungs within your rib cage. The axial framework also provides sites for the attachment of bones of the appendicular skeleton (eg, scapula), as well as muscles that move those bones (eg, serratus anterior). The musculoskeletal attachments thereby allow for movements that connect the two skeletons, for instance, scapular protraction (see Fig. 8.10). Movements proper to the axial skeleton occur throughout its regions including the vertebral column (eg, flexion of the back), head (eg, protraction of the jaw), and rib cage (eg, elevation of the ribs).

REGIONS OF THE AXIAL SKELETON

The regions related to the axial skeleton (Fig. 4.1) include
- The head is the most superior aspect of the axial skeleton—and the body—that sits on top of the neck. Its framework is formed by the skull. The neck, which includes the cervical spine, extends from the head to a base at the level of the clavicles anteriorly, and approximately the seventh cervical vertebra posteriorly.
- The back spans the posterior surface of the trunk, inferior to the neck and superior to the gluteal region. Its bony framework is primarily the vertebral column, which includes cervical, thoracic, lumbar, sacral, and coccygeal segments. It is commonly subcategorized into the middle back (related to the thoracic spine) and lower back (related to the lumbar spine). The sacrum sits below, between the pelvic ilia and on top the coccyx. The coccyx is the most distal portion of the axial skeleton, considered a vestigial tailbone that functions as an important attachment site for muscles, tendons, and ligaments, especially of the pelvic floor;

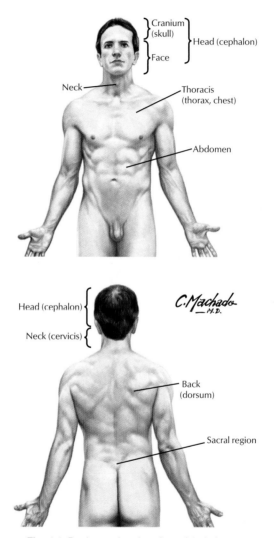

Fig. 4.1 Regions related to the axial skeleton.

it also assists in defecation (ie, extending with straining) and can serve as a balance mechanism when leaning back, for example, in a chair.

- The thorax is commonly considered the chest. Its region spans the superior thoracic aperture (the opening at the top of the rib cage) and the inferior thoracic aperture (the opening at the base of the rib cage that is closed by the diaphragm). The thoracic wall, a flexible cage of muscles and bones, binds the thorax anteriorly, posteriorly, and laterally. Place your hands on both sides of your torso to feel it. Within this wall is the thoracic cavity, which contains and protects important structures such as the heart, lungs, trachea, esophagus, diaphragm, vagus nerve, and phrenic nerves.
- The abdomen is generally defined as the lower portion of the trunk between the thorax and pelvis; many know it as the belly. This region houses many organs (eg, colon, kidneys, and spleen), which are protected by several layers of muscle and connective tissue. The muscles not only provide a protective sheath but also assist in many bodily functions such as respiration, childbirth, and defecation. Additionally, many of the muscles form an important part of the core (see "Movement: The Core" in Chapter 6).

BONES OF THE AXIAL SKELETON

- The skeletal framework of the axial skeleton includes the following bones (Fig. 4.2):
  - **Skull and Head**
    - **Calvaria, base (of cranium):** Fronal, temporal (2), parietal (2), occipital, sphenoid, ethmoid, and ossicles (malleus, incus, and stapes)
    - **Facial skeleton (of cranium):** Nasal (2), lacrimal (2), vomer (1), palatine (2), inferior nasal concha (2), zygomatic (2), and maxillae (2)
  - **Mandible**

- **Vertebral column**
  - **Neck:** Cervical vertebrae: C1 (atlas), C2 (axis), C3, C4, C5, C6, C7
  - **Back**
    - **Thoracic vertebrae:** T1, T2, T3, T4, T5, T6, T7, T8, T9, T10, T11, T12
    - **Lumbar vertebrae:** L1, L2, L3, L4, L5
  - **Sacrum:** One bone composed of five fused sacral vertebrae
  - **Coccyx:** One bone composed of three to five fused coccygeal vertebrae
- **Thorax**
  - **Ribs:** (true) 1 to 7, (false) 8 to 10, (floating) 11 to 12
  - **Sternum:** Composed of the manubrium, sternal body, and xiphoid process

MUSCLES OF THE AXIAL SKELETON

As is mentioned above, muscles that attach to the axial skeleton insert either on different regions of the axial skeleton (eg, the longissimus muscle, which is present in the thorax [thoracis], neck [cervicis], and head [capitis] regions) or on the appendicular skeleton (eg, the quadratus lumborum muscle, which connects the 12th rib, lumbar vertebrae, and pelvis). The muscles of the axial skeleton, then, have an expansive reach; they move the vertebral column, head, ribs, pelvis, and both sets of extremities (Tables 4.1 to 4.6 and Figs. 4.3 to 4.8). In addition to providing mobility, the region's muscles also contribute to stability (see "Movement: The Core" in Chapter 6). Of note, muscles of the pelvic floor are included in this chapter due to their connection with the core; in other references you may see them discussed in conjunction with the pelvic region.

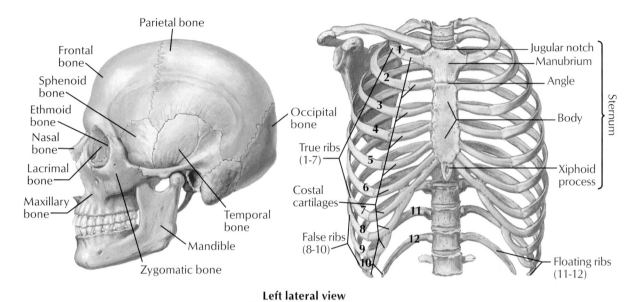

Parietal bone

Frontal bone

Sphenoid bone

Ethmoid bone

Nasal bone

Lacrimal bone

Maxillary bone

Occipital bone

True ribs (1-7)

Costal cartilages

False ribs (8-10)

Temporal bone

Mandible

Zygomatic bone

Jugular notch

Manubrium

Angle

Body

Xiphoid process

Sternum

Floating ribs (11-12)

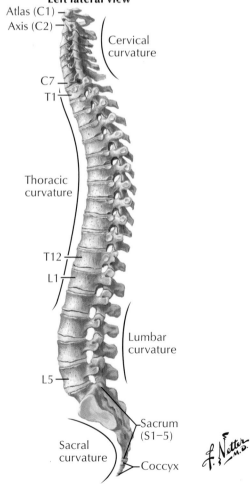

Left lateral view

Atlas (C1)

Axis (C2)

Cervical curvature

C7

T1

Thoracic curvature

T12

L1

Lumbar curvature

L5

Sacrum (S1–5)

Sacral curvature

Coccyx

Fig. 4.2 Bones of the axial skeleton.

TABLE 4.1   Muscles of the Head (Fig. 4.3)

Muscles	Comments
Mastication: Masseter, temporalis, lateral and medial pterygoids **Facial expression:** *Orbital group:* Orbicularis oculi, corrugator supercilii. *Nasal group:* Nasalis, procerus, depressor septi nasi. *Oral group*: Depressor anguli oris, depressor labii inferioris, mentalis, risorius, zygomaticus major and minor, levator labii superioris, levator labii superioris alaeque nasi, levator anguli oris, orbicularis oris, buccinator. *Other*: Occipitofrontalis, auricular (anterior, superior, posterior), platysma.	The muscles of the head can be grouped on the basis of function, innervation, and/or embryological derivation. The hyoid muscles, which are located in the neck, are also involved in mastication. In addition to the ones listed, other muscles intrinsic to the head include the extraocular muscles (move the eyeball and upper lid), muscles of the soft palate (elevate and depress the palate) and tongue (move and change the tongue's contour), and muscles of the middle ear (assist in the transmission of sound).

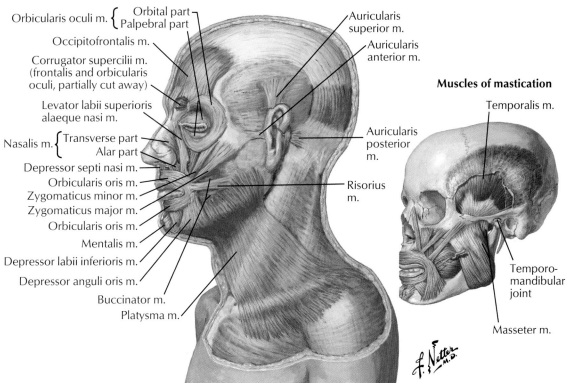

Fig. 4.3 Muscles of the head. (*Muscles not shown:* lateral and medial pterygoids, levator anguli oris.)

TABLE 4.2   Muscles of the Neck (Fig. 4.4)

Muscles	Comments
Posterior: Trapezius (upper fibers), levator scapulae, spinotransversales (splenius capitis and cervicis), erector spinae (iliocostalis cervicis, longissimus cervicis and capitis, spinalis cervicis and capitis), transversospinales (semispinalis cervicis and capitis, multifidus, rotatores cervicis). *Suboccipitals*: Rectus capitis posterior major and minor, obliquus capitis superior and inferior. **Anterior:** Sternocleidomastoid. *Prevertebral*: Longus capitis, longus colli, rectus capitis anterior and lateralis, scalenes (anterior, posterior, middle). *Suprahyoids*: mylohyoid, geniohyoid, stylohyoid, digastric. *Infrahyoids*: sternohyoid, omohyoid, sternothyroid, thyrohyoid.	Many of the posterior neck muscles are extensions of those in the back, indicated by their *cervicis* (neck) and *capitis* (head) denominations. Together, they stabilize, extend, laterally flex, and rotate the neck and head. The suboccipital muscles (Latin *sub*, "under"; *occiput*, "back of head") are intrinsic to the craniocervical region. On the anterior surface, most of the muscles act on the cervical spine to forward flex, laterally flex, or rotate the neck. The platysma is sometimes categorized here, as well, but is actually involved in facial expression. The hyoid muscles (Greek for "U-shaped") are located in the anterior traingle of the neck, in reference to the hyoid bone, either above (supra) or below (infra) it; they function in deglutition (swallowing).

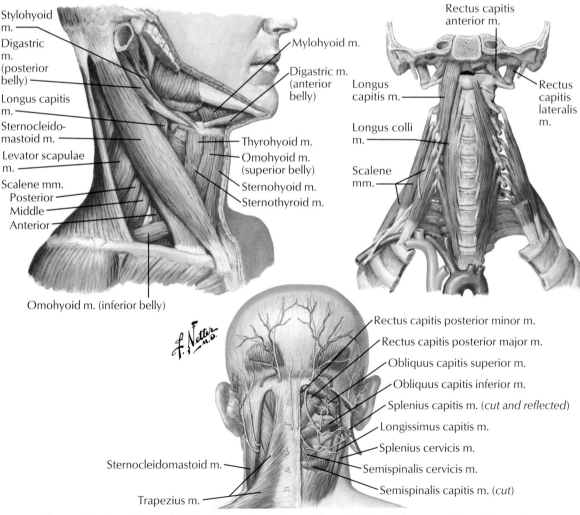

Fig. 4.4 Muscles of the neck. (*Muscles not shown:* iliocostalis cervicis, longissimus cervicis, spinalis cervicis and capitis, multifidus, rotatores cervicis, geniohyoid.)

TABLE 4.3 Muscles of the Back (Fig. 4.5)

Muscles	Comments
Superficial: Latissimus dorsi, trapezius, rhomboid major and minor, levator scapulae **Intermediate:** Serratus posterior superior and inferior **Deep:** *Erector spinae* (iliocostalis thoracis and lumborum, longissimus thoracis, spinalis thoracis). *Transversospinales* (semispinalis thoracis, multifidus, rotatores thoracis and lumborum). *Segmental muscles* (intertransversarii, interspinales, levatores costarum).	Of all the muscles located on the back, primarily the deep group moves and stabilizes it (with the exception of the levatores costarum muscles, which act on the ribs); they are considered the intrinsic muscles of the back. In contrast, the superficial muscles, which connect the trunk to the shoulder girdle, move the upper extremities, and the muscles of the intermediate group enable respiration. These two groups are thereby considered extrinsic muscles of the back.

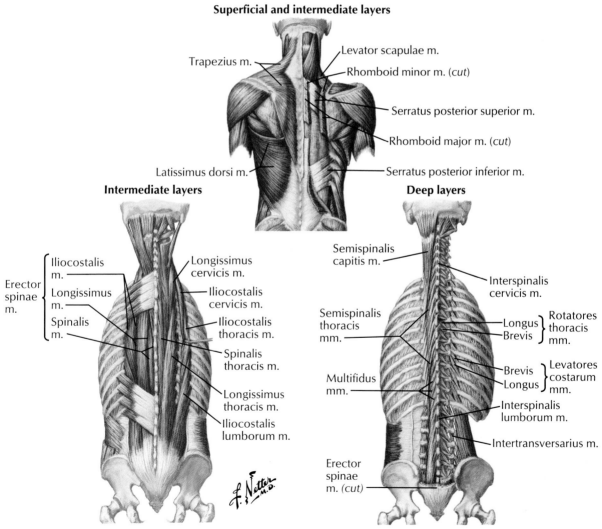

Superficial and intermediate layers

Trapezius m.

Levator scapulae m.

Rhomboid minor m. (*cut*)

Serratus posterior superior m.

Rhomboid major m. (*cut*)

Latissimus dorsi m.

Serratus posterior inferior m.

Intermediate layers

Erector spinae m. {
Iliocostalis m.
Longissimus m.
Spinalis m.
}

Longissimus cervicis m.

Iliocostalis cervicis m.

Iliocostalis thoracis m.

Spinalis thoracis m.

Longissimus thoracis m.

Iliocostalis lumborum m.

Deep layers

Semispinalis capitis m.

Interspinalis cervicis m.

Semispinalis thoracis mm.

Longus } Rotatores
Brevis } thoracis mm.

Brevis } Levatores
Longus } costarum mm.

Multifidus mm.

Interspinalis lumborum m.

Intertransversarius m.

Erector spinae m. (*cut*)

Fig. 4.5 Muscles of the back. (*Muscle not shown:* lumborum.)

TABLE 4.4 Muscles of the Thorax (Fig. 4.6)

Muscles	Comments
Proper: Diaphragm, intercostals (external, internal, innermost), subcostales, transversus thoracis **Thoracoappendicular:** *Anterior.* Pectoralis major and minor, subclavius, serratus anterior. *Posterior.* Trapezius, latissimus dorsi, levator scapulae, rhomboid major and minor.	The muscles of the thorax proper arise from and insert onto the rib cage; they are the main muscles of respiration. The thoracoappendicular muscles connect the thorax to the upper extremity and affect extrathoracic joints (eg, the pectoralis major—which arises from the rib cage, sternum, and clavicle, and inserts on the humerus—moves the shoulder joint). Of note, some of these muscles may also affect the intrathoracic joints, as accessory muscles of respiration. Other muscles of respiration found on the thorax, such as the levatores costarum and serratus posterior muscles, are categorized regionally with the muscles of the back.

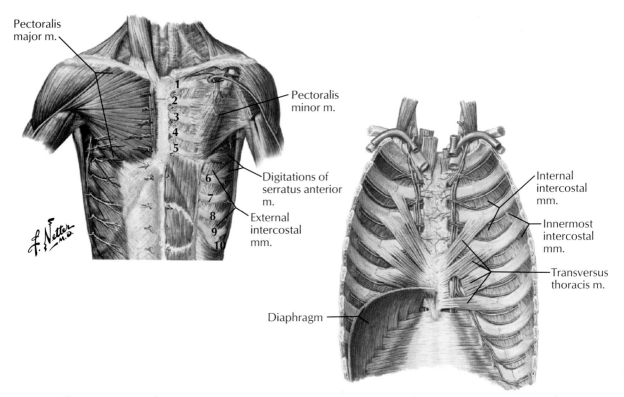

Fig. 4.6 Muscles of the thorax. (*Muscles not shown:* subcostales, subclavius, trapezius, latissimus dorsi, levator scapulae, rhomboid major and minor.)

TABLE 4.5	**Muscles of the Abdomen (Fig. 4.7)**
Muscles	**Comments**
Anterolateral wall: Rectus abdominis, external oblique, internal oblique, transversus abdominis, pyramidalis	The muscles of the anterolateral wall flex, laterally bend, and rotate the spine, as well as cover major organs, assist in respiration, and increase intraabdominal pressure during childbirth and urination/defecation.
Posterior wall: Iliacus, psoas major and minor, quadratus lumborum	The posterior wall muscles are ventral to the deep muscles of the back. Although they arise from and act on the vertebral column, they also impact the lower extremities. For instance, the iliacus and psoas muscles function together as the body's strongest hip flexor.

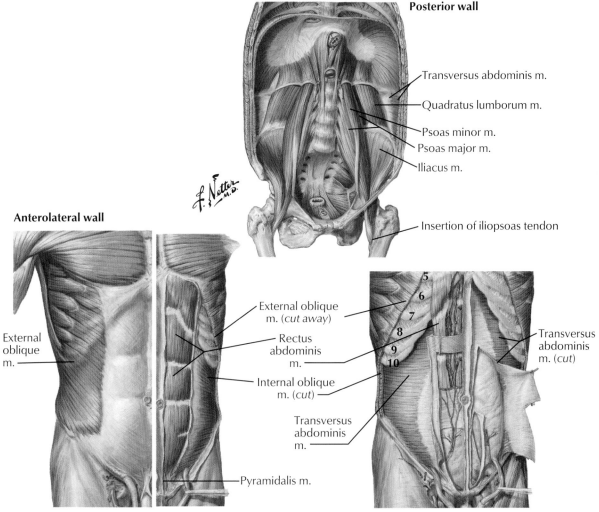

Fig. 4.7 Muscles of the abdomen.

TABLE 4.6   Muscles of the Pelvic Floor (Fig. 4.8)

Muscles	Comments
Pelvic diaphragm: (Ischio-) Coccygeus, levator ani (pubococcygeus, puborectalis, iliococcygeus) **Deep perineal pouch:** External urethral sphincter, compressor urethrae (women only), deep transverse perineal, sphincter urethrovaginalis	The muscles of the pelvic floor consists of those found in the pelvic diaphragm and deep perineal pouch. The pelvic diaphragm is known as the floor of the core because its muscles and fascia help stabilize the lower back and pelvis (see "Movement: The Core" in Chapter 6). The other muscles in the region act as sphincters and/or aid in sexual function as erectile tissue. Together, the pelvic floor muscles form a sling to support the pelvic organs so they can function correctly (eg, bladder, small intestines, uterus [women], prostate [men], and rectum). When they contract and relax, the muscles also assist in controlling bowel and bladder movements (Clinical Focus 4.1).

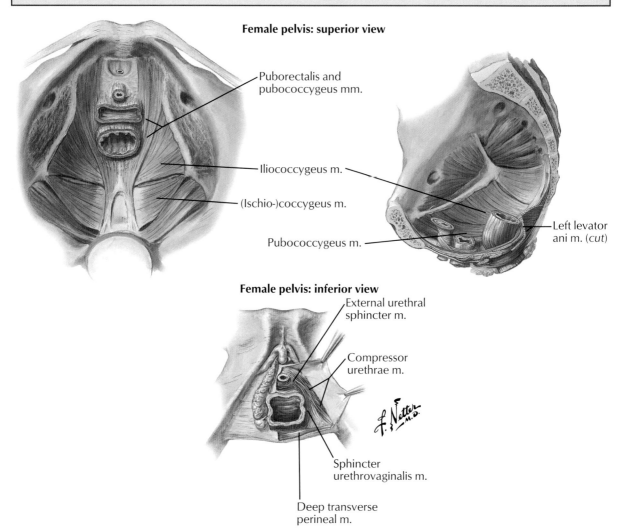

Female pelvis: superior view

Puborectalis and pubococcygeus mm.

Iliococcygeus m.

(Ischio-)coccygeus m.

Pubococcygeus m.

Left levator ani m. (cut)

Female pelvis: inferior view

External urethral sphincter m.

Compressor urethrae m.

Sphincter urethrovaginalis m.

Deep transverse perineal m.

Fig. 4.8 Muscles of the pelvic floor.

CLINICAL FOCUS 4.1   Pelvic Floor Dysfunction

Pelvic floor dysfunction (PFD) occurs when the pelvic muscles and connective tissue weaken or are injured, for instance, following childbirth or surgery or as a result of chronic coughing. One of the most common forms of PFD is pelvic organ prolapse, whereby the pelvic muscles and tissues can no longer support an organ, causing it to drop. In uterine prolapse, for example, the uterus may descend all the way into the vaginal opening. Bladder and bowel control problems can also occur, for instance, when the bladder or rectum shifts from its normal position; symptoms of bladder incontinence may include leakage of urine when coughing, sneezing, or jogging. Maintaining a healthy pelvic floor is therefore important not only to prevent PFD, but also to strengthen core musculature and enjoy a healthy sex life. To directly target these muscles, patients may be advised to try Kegel exercises, a practice that is akin to halting urination midstream. In addition, because the position of the pelvis can affect the function of the pelvic floor muscles, exercises such as the **Pilates Pelvic Tilts** (see Video 13.2) can play an important role in pelvic floor health.

SUMMARY

Overall, the muscles of the axial skeleton play an important role in stabilizing the skeleton, as well as mobilizing it. Stabilization of the vertebral column, in particular, is important because the column is the central structure around which most movements occur. The erector spinae group is one important set of spinal stabilizers, functioning to extend the entire spine and keep it erect (hence, its name). When these muscles are forced to work overtime or are misaligned (eg, when we spend excessive time sitting, slumping, and otherwise holding a forward flexed position), they become weakened and strained. For this reason, the paraspinals tend to play a role in chronic lower back pain. Of course, they do not act alone; other deep muscles, such as the transversospinales, intertransversarii, and interspinales muscles, are also known for their roles in stabilization.

Head

OVERVIEW

- The head is the most superior region of the body; it rests on the neck. It includes the face, sense organs, and brain.
- Its intrinsic articulations occur within the skull, between the temporal bone and mandible (the temporomandibular joint), the sutures of the skull (the suture joints), and the ossicles (the ossicular joints).
- Movements intrinsic to the region include mastication and motions of facial expression.
  - Craniocervical movements (eg, head and neck flexion) are discussed in Chapter 6, Neck and Back.
- Example exercise: **Yoga Lion's Pose** (see Video 5.1).

STRUCTURE AND FUNCTION

When you tap lightly on your head, you feel one solid bone. Your skull is actually composed of 22 bones (excluding the ossicles), however, and they are arranged in different regions. These regions evolved at different times, likely for different purposes. For example, the oldest parts of the skull, in evolutionary terms, are the bones (such as the occiput) in the lower region, known as the base. Many crucial openings (Latin, *foramina*) are found in the bones of the base; blood vessels pass through them, and nerves arising from the brain exit through them. Over time, as the human brain developed the bones surrounding it (such as the frontal and temporal bones) correspondingly grew and shifted. This is why, for instance, modern humans have a tall forehead. Finally, as our food supply became heartier, and thus more difficult to chew, the modern-day mandible and dentition came to the fore.

Today, the skull is commonly classified into two corresponding parts, the cranium and mandible.

Cranium

The cranium is the vault of the skull. It can be subdivided into an upper region (the calvaria), a base, and a lower anterior region (the facial skeleton).

Suture Joints

The bones forming the calvaria and base are the frontal (forehead) bone, temporal and parietal (headstand) bones, and occipital, sphenoid, and ethmoid bones. These flat bones are connected by strong suture joints, such as the joint between the occipital and parietal bones (see Fig. 5.1A). A suture joint is a fibrous type of solid joint used in areas that require great strength and protection (in this case, the skull is protecting the brain). Although suture joints afford little or no movement for the bones that they connect in adult life, their connections do allow for movement as an infant is developing. In fact, their early malleability allows a baby's head to fit through the birth canal, without damaging the brain. Subsequently, as the brain grows and develops, it may take up to 2 years for the sutures to close.

Ossicular Joints

Lodged within the temporal bone on each side of the head are three, small bones: the malleus, incus, and stapes (Latin for "hammer," "anvil," and "stirrup," names that indicate their respective shapes) (see Fig. 5.1B). Along with the tympanic membrane, the bones are located in the middle ear and function primarily to transmit sound waves to the brain (where they are processed into familiar words, songs, and other sounds). Although the bones

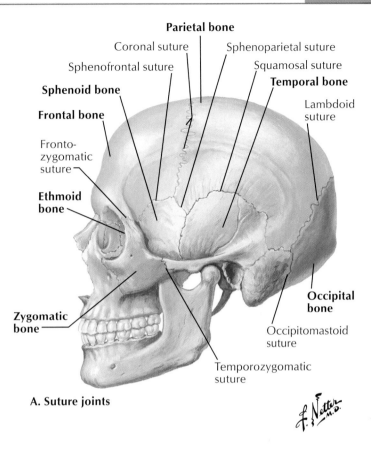

Parietal bone

Coronal suture

Sphenofrontal suture

Sphenoparietal suture

Squamosal suture

Temporal bone

Sphenoid bone

Lambdoid
suture

Frontal bone

Fronto-
zygomatic
suture

**Ethmoid
bone**

**Occipital
bone**

**Zygomatic
bone**

Occipitomastoid
suture

Temporozygomatic
suture

A. Suture joints

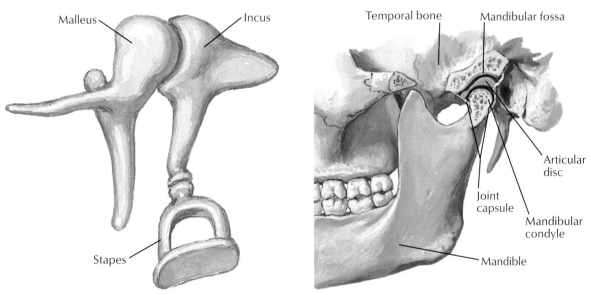

Malleus   Incus

Temporal bone   Mandibular fossa

Articular
disc

Joint
capsule

Mandibular
condyle

Stapes

Mandible

B. Ossicular joints

C. Temporomandibular joint

Fig. 5.1 Joints of the head.

can be visualized by the naked eye, they are very small; indeed, the stapes is the smallest bone in the body. Not surprisingly, these small bones are accompanied by the two smallest striated muscles in the body, the tensor tympani and stapedius muscles. Despite the size of these bones, the joints connecting them are synovial, just like the joints found in larger structures of the body, such as the knee and shoulder. As with their larger counterparts, the ossicular joints are susceptible to injury; for instance, when joint damage and inflammation occur due to rheumatoid arthritis, hearing impairment may also occur.

Facial Skeleton

When you see a loved one and your face "lights up," your muscles of facial expression are moving to indicate happiness. The zygomatic major muscle, for instance, is elevating the corners of the mouth upward into a smile. Although there are no joints that enable the movement, the facial bones provide a foundation for it. These bones, which give your face its basic structure include the maxilla (the upper jaw), nasal bone (the bridge of the nose), zygomatic bone (the cheekbone), and lacrimal bone (a fragile bone of the orbital socket) (see Chapter 4, Regional Overview of the Axial Skeleton). Their structure also supports the muscles involved in facial expression (Table 5.1).

Mandible

The mandible, or lower jawbone, is not typically considered part of the facial skeleton or cranium (see Fig.

TABLE 5.1   Muscles of Facial Expression and Their Actions (see Fig. 4.3).

Muscle	Action
Orbital Group	
Orbicularis oculi	Eyelids close
Corrugator supercilii	Eyebrows draw medially and downward, forming vertical wrinkles above nose (ie, a frown)
Nasal Group	
Nasalis	Nasal apertures open and close (ie, flaring nostrils)
Procerus	Medial angle of eyebrows draws down, producing transverse wrinkles over bridge of nose (ie, a frown)
Depressor septi	Nose pulls inferiorly (ie, flaring nostrils)
Oral Group	
Depressor anguli oris	Corners of mouth draw down and laterally (ie, a frown)
Depressor labii inferioris	Lower lip draws down and laterally
Mentalis	Lower lip raises and protrudes, as skin on chin wrinkles (ie, helps mouth drink from cup)
Risorius	Corners of mouth retract (ie, a grin)
Zygomaticus major	Corners of mouth draw upward and laterally (ie, helps one smile)
Zygomaticus minor	Upper lip drawns upward (ie, helps one smile)
Levator labii superioris	Upper lip raises; nostrils open; nasolabial furrow formed
Levator labii superioris alaque nasi	Upper lip raises and nostrils open (ie, assists in flaring nostrils)
Levator anguli oris	Corners of mouth raise; nasolabial furrow forms
Orbicularis oris	Lips close and protrude (ie, helps whistle)
Buccinator	Cheeks press against the teeth; compresses distended cheeks (ie, helps blow out a mouthful of air)
Other Muscles	
Occipitofrontalis	Forehead wrinkles; eyebrows raise; scalp draws backward
Auricular (anterior, superior, posterior)	Ears elevate and draw upward, forward, and backward (Box 5.1)
Platysma	Skin of neck tenses

BOX 5.1 **Wiggling Your Ears**

Although they are not located directly on the face, the three auricular muscles that surround the ear are considered muscles of facial expression. Some researchers think that their movements, which wiggle the ears, may have helped with sound localization, as similar muscles do in many mammals (think about how a cat cocks her ear toward even the faintest noise). Today, however, these muscles are considered relatively unimportant. They are nonetheless skeletal muscles innervated by branches of the facial nerve (cranial nerve [CN] VII, which innervates the muscles of facial expression). Some people, therefore, can move their ears naturally, and others can do so with a little practice.

CLINICAL FOCUS 5.1
Temporomandibular Joint Disorder

The temporomandibular joint (TMJ) is the largest synovial joint of the skull, permitting the jaw to move in ways that facilitate everyday activities such as talking, chewing, and yawning. Like its synovial counterparts in the extremities, the TMJ is subject to wear and tear; in fact, temporomandibular disorder (TMD) is one of the most common causes of facial pain. Despite its prevalence, the etiology of TMD is multifactorial, including trauma to the head (eg, whiplash), severe tension in the suboccipital muscles, repetitive microtrauma (eg, grinding of the teeth), and/or structural dispositions (eg, malocclusion of the jaw). The classic symptom is a radiating pain that emanates from the jaw; other symptoms include tightness of the neck muscles, headaches, and restricted jaw function, all of which are likely to increase during times of stress. Because individuals with TMD may also present with a fixed, head-forward position (see Practice What You Preach 5.1), symptoms may be eased by properly balancing the head and neck muscles with the **Yoga Cobra Pose** (see Video 6.2) and the **Pilates Head Nods**. Decreasing one's overall stress level, by doing breath work or meditation, can also help. Manual therapy of the musculature and ligaments around the joint may further relieve symptoms.

5.1). Like the skull, the mandible appears to be a single bone, but it is actually a composite of two bones that fuse very early on in life. It is the largest and strongest of the facial bones, houses your lower set of teeth, and hosts attachment sites for the many muscles responsible for moving the jaw. It is very mobile, which is important for its role in the temporomandibular joint.

Temporomandibular Joint

The temporomandibular joint (TMJ) is a synovial hinge joint formed between the mandible and temporal bones; the condyle of the mandible projects into the mandibular fossa of the temporal bone, with an articular disc that divides the joint into two sections (superior and inferior) joint cavities (see Fig. 5.1C). Everyone has two TMJs, one on each side of the face. Like most synovial joints, the TMJ has supportive connective tissue structures such as ligaments (eg, temporomandibular ligament), a fibrous capsule, and the aforementioned articular disc, which cushions the strong and repetitive joint motions. Unlike other synovial joints, its articulating surfaces are not covered by hyaline cartilage; they are instead covered by fibrocartilage, which absorbs force better than its hyaline counterpart. This makes the joint less distensible but better able to bear repetitive stress (ie, so you can chew gum). Indeed, the TMJs are two of the most continuously used joints in the body, enabling the jaw to elevate, depress, protract, retract, and translate side to side (see Fig. 5.2). These movements form the basis of mastication, or your ability to chew, tear, and grind food with your teeth. Although well built for endurance, the joint can be subject to aches and pains associated with repetitive stress (given

how frequently you masticate, swallow, speak, and yawn) (Clinical Focus 5.1).

MOVEMENTS

Most of the movements of your head are guided by the sense organs of the head, that is, the eyes, ears, nose, mouth, and skin. These organs provide different types of information to help you interact safely and smartly with your environment: Your eyes, for instance, help detect a car coming down the street; your ears hear a cry for help; your nose smells smoke; and your tongue tastes rancid food that needs to be thrown out. It is very helpful, then, that the head is able to rotate almost 180 degrees from side to side to register the greatest number of impressions (Box 5.2). This rotational movement—in addition to flexion and extension—is enabled by the cervical spine and its articulation with the occiput, as discussed in Chapter 6, Neck and Back. The following section discusses movements intrinsic to the head, which occur at the TMJ: elevation, depression, protrusion, retrusion, and lateral excursion (Fig. 5.2). Together, these

BOX 5.2   A Balanced Body

Movement requires components like muscles, bones, and nerves. Another component, balance, is equally important. In a gym or movement studio, "finding your balance" is typically mentioned in relationship to your core (see Chapter 6), foot placement, or as a cue to find a visual focal point. Balance, however, actually begins with the higher command centers that keep you coordinated and upright in the first place, including the brain, inner ear, and cervical muscles. These command centers, complex in themselves, are integrated through an intricate system of neural communications, fluid hemodynamics, and muscle movements.

For instance, the brain needs signals from the inner ear to interpret features of the environment and adjust the position of your head. The inner ear includes a bony labyrinth that contains the cochlea (the organ for hearing) and the semicircular canals. These canals are filled with fluid and are connected to nerve cells that report movement to the brain. This intricate system enables the brain to detect subtle shifts of fluid position, which, in turn, determine how your head should be positioned for optimal body balance. The

third balance command center is made up of the cervical muscles (eg, rectus capitis posterior minor), which position your head in response to signals from the inner ear. Working in tandem, these muscles facilitate a matrix of movements that refine the head's position in order to achieve total body coordination.

Conversely, lack of balance may occur when the balance command centers are deregulated by external or internal factors. External deregulation may occur when your muscles are inappropriately engaged, as when you shake your head quickly and then try to walk. Internal deregulation may occur when the delicate fluids and nerve cells within the inner ear are adversely affected, as after drinking too much alcohol. With dysfunction of the centers, the head position is disturbed and so, therefore, are coordination of trunk and limb movements. So the next time you are finding your balance in exercise class, consider not only the engagement of your core and the position of your feet but also how you are moving and using your head.

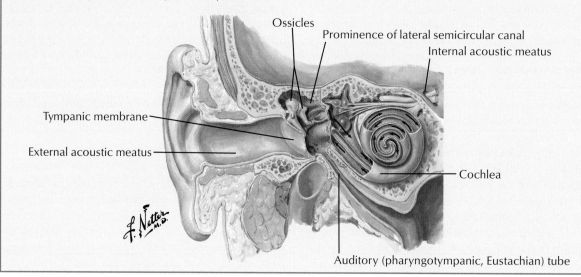

movements enable mastication, in addition to all the daily activities for which your jaw is used.

Depression and Elevation

Try getting a spoonful of soup into a closed mouth to appreciate depression of the mandible (see Fig. 5.2A). Depression is the movement that opens the mouth, and it is needed whether you are eating, yawning, speaking,

or screaming. An adult mouth can be opened an average of 2 inches, or the width of three adult knuckles (measured between the incisal edges of the upper and lower front teeth). Elevation is the movement that subsequently closes the mouth (see Fig. 5.2A). During these movements, the TMJ experiences a complex combination of rotation and translation between the mandibular condyle and fossa; additionally, to fully depress the mandible and open the

A. Depression/Elevation

B. Protrusion/Retraction

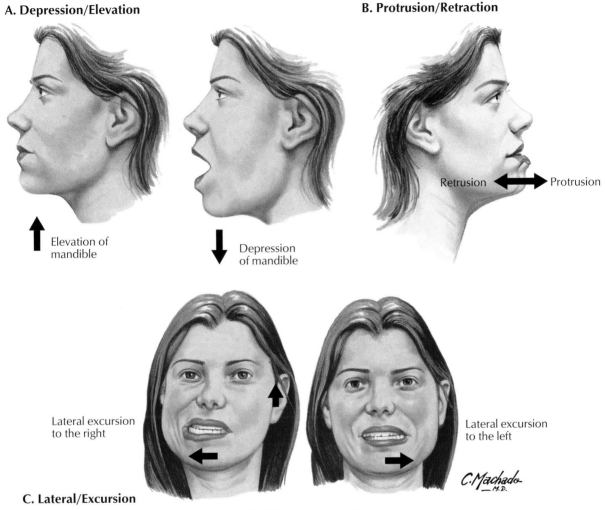

Elevation of
mandible

Depression
of mandible

Retrusion ←→ Protrusion

Lateral excursion
to the right

Lateral excursion
to the left

C. Machado
— M.D.

C. Lateral/Excursion

Fig. 5.2 Jaw movements.

mouth, extreme anterior translation (protrusion) is also required. Full depression and elevation occur in different phases (similar to the multiple phases involved in full abduction of the arm); the articular disc is an active component throughout, helping guide the jaw's motion while decreasing stress on the articular surfaces (Practice What You Preach 5.1).

Protrusion and Retrusion

If you were to mimic a bulldog, the first thing you would do is protrude your jaw, so that it would move anteriorly. Protrusion also helps depression open the mouth as wide as possible. Retrusion is the action opposite from protrusion (see Fig. 5.2B). It returns the jaw posteriorly, helping

---

PRACTICE WHAT YOU PREACH 5.1
A Head Above the Rest

Look around and you'll notice many individuals sitting at their desks or walking down the street with their heads protruding. This forward-head posture involves a flexed upper thoracic and lower cervical spine, with an extended craniocervical region. In such cases, the mandible is also affected and is pulled in the direction of retrusion and depression. So, when you find yourself slouching and act to straighten the posture of your head, neck, and shoulders, don't forget your mandible. Actively realign it into a neutral, closed (but not clenched) position to properly reposition your entire head.

to close a widely opened mouth. During protrusion and retrusion, the mandibular condyle and articular disc move anteriorly and posteriorly, respectively, relative to the mandibular fossa.

Lateral Excursion

To relax a clenched jaw, you may move it from side to side. This motion is lateral excursion, which can occur to the left or to the right (see Fig. 5.2C). The movement primarily involves a side-to-side translation of the mandibular condyle and articular disc within the mandibular fossa, accompanied by a very slight rotation. It is particularly important in grinding food between the teeth.

SUMMARY

Although the two TMJs work together for jaw mobility, they do so asymmetrically—one side is more dominant (exerting a greater force) than the other, similar to having a dominant arm when throwing a ball. While the mandible and temporal bones are the joint articulators, they are assisted by several surrounding bones, such as the maxillae and zygomatic, sphenoid, and hyoid bones, which aid the structure and function of the TMJ. For instance, the

sphenoid hosts attachment sites for the pterygoid muscles. The primary muscles that move the TMJ are innervated by the mandibular nerve, a division of CN V.

MUSCLES

See Fig. 5.3.

Movement	Muscles
Elevation	Masseter
	Temporalis
	Medial pterygoid
Depression	Lateral pterygoid
	Suprahyoids
	Infrahyoids (stabilize the hyoid bone to assist the suprahyoids)
Protrusion	Lateral pterygoid
Retrusion	Temporalis
Lateral excursion	Masseter
	Temporalis
	Medial pterygoid
	Lateral pterygoid
Deglutition	Suprahyoids
	Infrahyoids
	See Table 4.2.

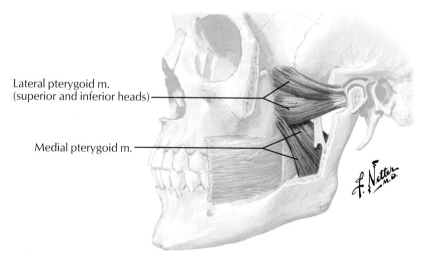

Lateral pterygoid m. (superior and inferior heads)

Medial pterygoid m.

Fig. 5.3 Muscles that move the jaw (see Fig. 4.3 for masseter, temporalis).

Moving Anatome Exercise
Mandible Depression: Yoga Lion's Pose (Simhasana)

See Fig. 5.4 and Video 5.1.

Once you feel comfortable making the "funny face" in this pose, make some of your childhood funny faces and note how most of them incorporate movements of the mandible.

- Starting position: Kneeling on the floor, sitting on your heels, toes extended. Hands are on your thighs, with palms facing down and fingers extended.
- Inhale deeply through your nose, filling your chest with air.
- Exhale forcefully and make a "*ha*" sound while:
  - Opening your mouth wide and sticking your tongue out and down toward your chin, as far as it will go.
  - Opening your eyes wide and gazing upward toward the midbrow.
  - Pressing your palms against your thighs with elbows extended.
- Repeat three times.
- Ending position: Kneeling, with a neutral face.

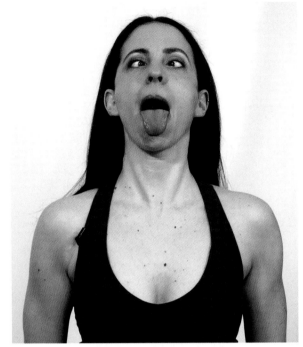

Fig. 5.4 Mandible depression: **Yoga Lion's Pose (Simhasana)** (see Video 5.1).

6

Neck and Back

OVERVIEW

- The vertebral column is composed of 33 vertebrae divided into five regions: cervical, thoracic, lumbar, sacral, and coccygeal.
- Two main categories of joints exist in the vertebral column: stabilizers (symphysial joints) and mobilizers (facet joints, atlantoaxial and occipital joints, and costovertebral and costotransverse joints).
- Movements of the vertebral column include flexion, extension, lateral flexion, and rotation.
- Example exercises:
  - Flexion (**Pilates Roll Up**, Video 6.1)
  - Extension (**Yoga Cobra Pose**, Video 6.2)
  - Lateral flexion (**Yoga Extended Side Angle Pose**, Video 6.3)
  - Rotation (**Pilates Spine Twist**, Video 6.4)

STRUCTURE AND FUNCTION OF THE VERTEBRAL COLUMN

What does the phrase "have a strong backbone" mean to you? In common parlance, it describes a person who demonstrates qualities such as fortitude and determination, particularly in the face of a challenge. That same definition rings true on an anatomical level. Each day, your backbone (vertebral column) dutifully works against gravity to serve as scaffolding for your upright torso, while it also protects the spinal cord encased within it. In addition to being strong, the vertebral column is impressively flexible. It enables the torso to move through a wide range of motions while simultaneously supporting the mobility of the upper and lower limbs. Given the duality of its work, the vertebral column must maintain a balance between stability and mobility; otherwise, problems develop, such as spinal stenosis (in which an excess of rigidity decreases mobility; see Clinical Focus 6.2) or intervertebral disc herniation (in which too much flexibility leads to a loss of stability; see Clinical Focus 6.1).

What allows for the dual function of the vertebral column? It is the column's multifaceted structure. Composed of 33 individual vertebrae, the vertebral column is organized into five segments: cervical, thoracic, lumbar, sacral, and coccygeal (Fig. 6.1). The cervical region is often referred to as the neck, the thoracic, lumbar and sacral segments collectively as the back, and the coccyx as the tailbone. The cervical spine contains 7 vertebrae, the thoracic spine has 12 (1 to articulate with each of the 12 ribs), the lumbar spine has 5, the sacral spine has 5, and the coccyx contains 3 to 5. Each bony segment exhibits unique characteristics that not only determine its gross appearance but also its range of movement (Box 6.1).

Despite their regional differences, vertebrae have many similarities. A typical vertebra has two parts, a body and an arch. Two pedicles attach the vertebral body and arch; two laminae form the roof of each arch. Protruding from the arch of each vertebra are three types of processes (Latin *process*, "outgrowth"): spinous, transverse, and articular (Fig. 6.2). These processes provide attachment sites for muscles of the back and neck, as well as articular surfaces at which adjacent vertebrae interlock. A typical vertebra articulates with a neighboring vertebra via six joints: four synovial (two above, two below) and two symphysial (one above, one below). These articulations allow the vertebral column, as a whole, to perform its functions as both a stabilizer and a mobilizer by (1) protecting the spinal cord and nerves encased within its central canal (vertebral foramen), (2) supporting the body's weight and posture, (3) providing an axis around which the body can move, and (4) assisting in locomotion

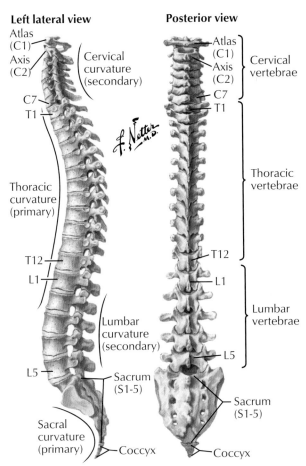

Left lateral view

Atlas (C1)
Axis (C2)

Cervical curvature (secondary)

C7
T1

Thoracic curvature (primary)

T12
L1

Lumbar curvature (secondary)

L5

Sacrum (S1-5)

Sacral curvature (primary)

Coccyx

Posterior view

Atlas (C1)
Axis (C2)
C7
T1

Cervical vertebrae

Thoracic vertebrae

T12
L1

Lumbar vertebrae

L5

Sacrum (S1-5)

Coccyx

Fig. 6.1. Regions and curvatures of the vertebral column.

from one place to another. Regionally, the articulations allow the cervical, thoracic, and lumbar spines to move freely; the sacral and coccygeal segments remain relatively immobile because their connecting joints are fused (Figs. 6.3 and 6.4). All of these articulations fall into two main categories: stabilizers and mobilizers.

The Stabilizers: Symphysial Joints

The stabilizers are cartilaginous joints known as symphyses; they are also referred to as intervertebral joints. Each symphysial joint connects two adjacent vertebral bodies with a fibrocartilaginous intervertebral disc sandwiched between them (Fig. 6.5). Only slight movement is permitted at this cartilaginous joint. Its main roles are to bear weight, absorb shock, and provide stability (Box 6.2 and Clinical Focus 6.1).

The Mobilizers
Facet Joints

You can sit up, do a backbend, and twist thanks to 24 pairs of mobile zygapophyseal joints, commonly known as facet joints. These joints connect the superior articular facet of one vertebral arch with the inferior articular facet of the vertebral arch above it. This synovial articulation between two smooth surfaces allows for a gliding

---

BOX 6.1 Regional Differences

Despite their similarities, vertebrae exhibit different compositions and functions. For example, the cervical vertebrae provide a throughway for major vessels of the head and neck, and thus contain distinctive holes, called foramina, through which these structures pass. The thoracic vertebrae articulate with the rib cage and, therefore, have specific articular facets just for the ribs. Moving inferiorly the vertebral bodies become progressively larger in order to bear the body's increasing weight burden, culminating in the sizable lumbar vertebral bodies. Spinous processes also differ from vertebra to vertebra; some are bifid (eg, split in two), some are long, some are short, and some are rudimentary; in some cases, the processes are absent (see Fig. 6.2).

BOX 6.2 Intervertebral Disc

Your vertebral column bears a lot of weight every time you move, even when you stand. If your bones had to handle this load alone, they would likely deteriorate quickly. Thankfully, you have intervertebral (IV) discs, which are round, gel-like cushions, softening every step you take.

Commonly likened to a jelly doughnut, an IV disc has two layers: an inner gelatinous mass (the nucleus pulposus) and an outer fibrous casing (the anulus fibrosus). The content of the nucleus pulposus is mostly water, affording it the ability to act as a modified hydraulic shock absorber every time the spine moves. The water composition decreases with age, culminating in a loss of vertical height. The tougher anulus fibrosus surrounds the inner pulposus with fibrocartilaginous concentric layers, increasing the disc's shock absorbing capability. In addition to shock absorption, the two components of the IV disc provide intervertebral stability and an axis of rotation for spinal movement.

See also Clinical Focus 6.1.

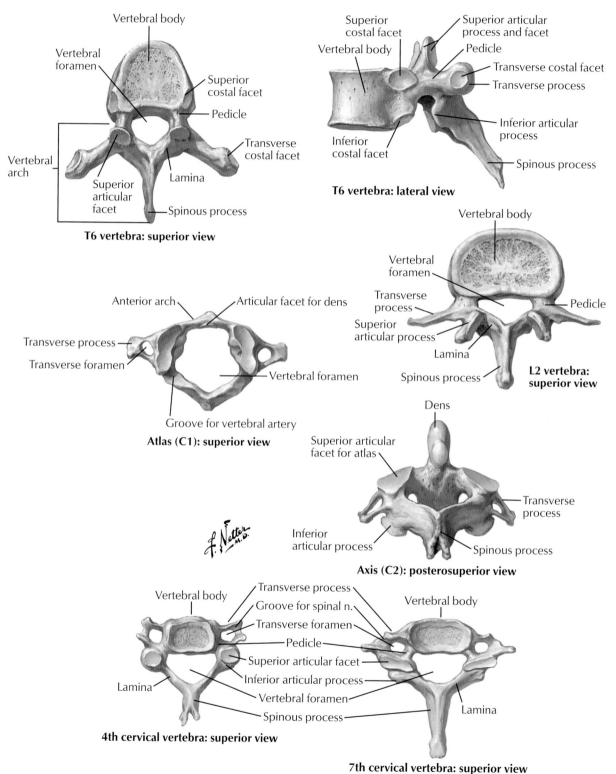

T6 vertebra: superior view

Vertebral body

Vertebral foramen

Superior costal facet

Pedicle

Transverse costal facet

Vertebral arch

Superior articular facet

Lamina

Spinous process

T6 vertebra: lateral view

Superior costal facet

Vertebral body

Superior articular process and facet

Pedicle

Transverse costal facet

Transverse process

Inferior costal facet

Inferior articular process

Spinous process

Atlas (C1): superior view

Anterior arch

Articular facet for dens

Transverse process

Transverse foramen

Vertebral foramen

Groove for vertebral artery

L2 vertebra: superior view

Vertebral body

Vertebral foramen

Transverse process

Pedicle

Superior articular process

Lamina

Spinous process

Axis (C2): posterosuperior view

Dens

Superior articular facet for atlas

Transverse process

Inferior articular process

Spinous process

4th cervical vertebra: superior view

Vertebral body

Transverse process

Groove for spinal n.

Transverse foramen

Pedicle

Superior articular facet

Inferior articular process

Vertebral foramen

Spinous process

Lamina

Vertebral body

7th cervical vertebra: superior view

Lamina

Fig. 6.2. Examples of vertebrae.

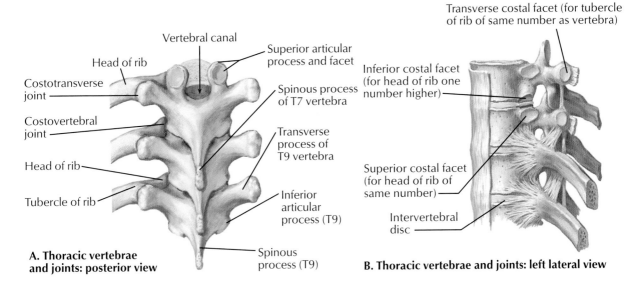

A. Thoracic vertebrae and joints: posterior view

B. Thoracic vertebrae and joints: left lateral view

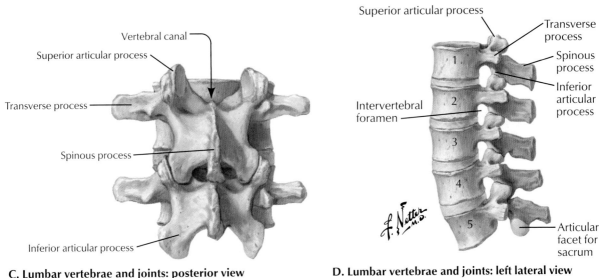

C. Lumbar vertebrae and joints: posterior view

D. Lumbar vertebrae and joints: left lateral view

Fig. 6.3. Facet and costovertebral joints.

motion; the amount of motion allowed is determined by the shape and orientation of the facets, which differ throughout the vertebral column. For example, turn your head to the right. Now, see if you can rotate your lower back as far to the right without moving your pelvis. You probably cannot. The greater range of motion of the neck compared with the more limited range of motion of the lower back is primarily due to the differing orientation

of the facets found in the cervical and lumbar spines, respectively.

Atlantooccipital and Atlantoaxial Joints

The atlantooccipital and atlantoaxial joints are specialized joint structures that facilitate nuanced positioning of the head, so you can see, smell, and hear your environment, all while maintaining equilibrium. The atlantooccipital

CLINICAL FOCUS 6.1   Intervertebral Disc Bulge and Herniation

As bodies age, so do their intervertebral discs and the ligaments protecting them; for instance, the nucleus pulposus dries out, the anulus fibrosus turns brittle, and the posterior longitudinal ligament (which buttresses the posterior edge of the disc) weakens. Together, these changes can lead to increased risks of disc bulges and herniations, two common injuries that involve a displacement of a disc (or some part of it) from its intervertebral "home." A disc bulge is a generalized outpouching of a disc's outer edges (ie, the whole disc appears swollen). In contrast, a disc herniation is defined as a localized displacement (ie, a focal protrusion) of disc material. Whether bulged or herniated, a degenerated disc may provoke a cascade of problems, including microtears and muscle spasms, plus bony changes of the spine to compensate for developing instability; the term degenerative disc disease encompasses all of these symptoms.

Other causes such as trauma, can also incite disc injury, but degeneration is the most common. Both disc herniations and bulges are frequently found in the lumbar and cervical spines and can either be silent or symptomatic, with the latter often presenting as localized back pain and radiating neuropathic pain if there is impingement on a nerve root and/or the spinal cord. Physical rehabilitation of disc herniations focuses on strengthening and stabilizing the core, as well as facilitating movements that lessen and centralize symptoms (eg, a modified **Yoga Plank Pose** [see Video 8.4] on your knees) and avoiding movements that exacerbate or peripheralize symptoms. Simultaneous flexion and rotation of the spine (eg, abdominal sit-ups with rotation), for example, would likely be contraindicated, because this movement increases stress on the intervertebral discs of the lumbar spine and could aggravate symptoms.

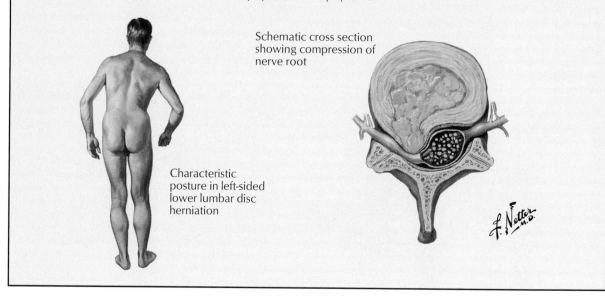

Schematic cross section showing compression of nerve root

Characteristic posture in left-sided lower lumbar disc herniation

joint is formed between the concave superior articular facets of the atlas (C1) and the convex condyles of the occipital bone; this convex-concave fit confers an inherent stability to the joint. Generally, the joint permits flexion and extension of the craniocervical region. The atlantoaxial joint is a complex of joints between the atlas and axis (C2) (see Fig. 6.4). In addition to a pair of lateral facet joints, there is a median joint featuring the dens of C2 protruding into a combination of the transverse ligament and anterior arch of the atlas; together, the complex plays a primary role in craniocervical rotation.

Together, the atlantooccipital and atlantoaxial joints confer extra range of motion to an already mobile cervical spine (the most mobile part of the vertebral column). See this for yourself as you shake your head "yes" and "no." The mobility of these joints, however, is confined to a safe range secondary to surrounding structures such as the atlantooccipital membranes, which prevent excessive hyperflexion and hyperextension, and the atlantoaxial ligaments, which prevent excessive rotation. Otherwise, these vertebrae, like the others, would naturally keep moving in the direction of least bony resistance.

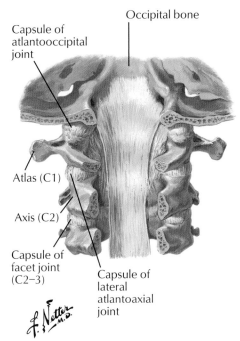

Occipital bone

Capsule of
atlantooccipital
joint

Atlas (C1)

Axis (C2)

Capsule of
facet joint
(C2–3)

Capsule of
lateral
atlantoaxial
joint

Fig. 6.4. Atlantoaxial and atlantooccipital joints. Upper part of vertebral canal with spinous processes and parts of vertebral arches removed to expose ligaments on posterior vertebral bodies: posterior view.

Costovertebral and Costotransverse Joints

The thoracic spine articulates with 12 pairs of ribs (Latin *costo*, "rib") (see Fig. 6.3). The costovertebral joint connects the head of a rib to a pair of costal facets that span adjacent vertebrae. The costotransverse joint connects the tubercle of a rib (usually 1–10) to the costal facet on the transverse process of a related vertebra. Through these connections, the thoracic spine and ribs form the posterior thoracic cage, helping to provide a sturdy structure for (1) protection of vital organs enclosed within (ie, heart, lungs) and (2) attachments of muscles that act on the craniocervical and appendicular regions. At the cost of size and strength, however, comes mobility, as the ribcage limits the range of motion of the thoracic spine. Thoracic movements are not large, but they are some of the most frequent movements you make each day, because the ribs elevate and depress every time you breathe.

MOVEMENT

The vertebral column is one of the more mobile structures of the human body. It can flex, laterally flex, extend, and

rotate (Fig. 6.6). Each movement is the sum of relatively small motions between individual vertebrae. Better yet, each segment of the back has its own capacity to engage in these movements simultaneously, so that you can flex your thoracic and lumbar spines to clean up spilled milk on the floor while you extend your cervical spine to see if you missed any drops (Box 6.3).

Key factors determine how each spinal segment moves. They include (1) the shape, orientation, and capsule tension of the facet joints, (2) the thickness, elasticity, and compressibility of intervertebral discs, and (3) the condition and actions of surrounding muscles and ligaments. These factors determine the range of motion in different segments of the spine, allowing for expansive mobility in some areas (eg, the cervical spine) and limited movement in others (eg, the thoracic spine). Regardless of their extent, the presence of limitations to movement is central to the overall stabilization of the spinal column and the prevention of injury (Practice What You Preach 6.1).

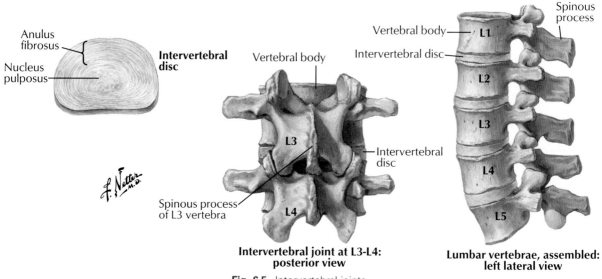

Fig. 6.5. Intervertebral joints.

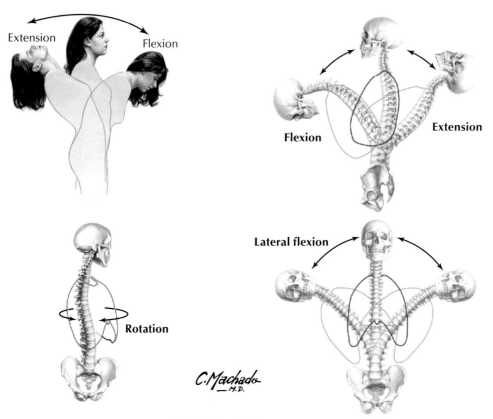

Fig. 6.6. Vertebral movements.

FLEXION

Back Flexion

Many individuals have a goal of touching their toes, and forward flexion of the back turns this dream into reality. Flexion brings the anterior surfaces of two vertebral bodies closer together. The inferior facets of each superior vertebra slide upward against the superior facets of each vertebra below it; this, in turn, allows the superior vertebral body to tilt anteriorly atop of the intervening intervertebral disc. As a result, the disc is compressed in the front and opened in the back. The amount of flexion allowed is determined by facet orientation. For example, the almost vertical facet orientation in the lumbar spine allows for a considerable degree of flexion. General factors limiting flexion include tension provided by facet joint capsules, posterior spinal ligaments, and the extensor muscles of the back. In the thoracic spine, flexion is also limited by the presence of the costovertebral and costotransverse joints (Clinical Focus 6.2).

Head and Neck Flexion

Go ahead, give an affirming nod. Your ability to concur with a true statement is due, in part, to head and neck flexion. Head flexion occurs at the atlantooccipital joint as the head, at the convex occipital condyles, tilts anteriorly upon the concave articular facets of the atlas. Some flexion also occurs at the atlantoaxial joint as the ring-shaped atlas pivots forward atop the axis. Most elements of flexion, however, happen throughout the remaining intracervical articulations, with the lower region (C4-C7) initiating the movement as the inferior articular facets of the superior vertebrae slide superiorly and anteriorly relative to the superior facets of the inferior vertebrae.

Try **Moving AnatoME** with **Pilates Roll Up** (Video 6.1). Slowly flex forward at the head and neck, followed by the back. Notice how even though you are doing the same movement throughout the exercise, you are able to isolate flexion at each region and observe how differently each region's movement feels.

Approximate Range of Motion

- Back: 85 degrees (thoracic = 35 degrees, lumbar = 50 degrees)
- Head and neck: 50 degrees

Muscles and Innervation

See Fig. 6.7.

Muscle	Nerve
Back	
Rectus abdominis	T6-T12 (ventral rami)
External oblique	T6-T12 (ventral rami) and subcostal nerve
Internal oblique	T6-L1 (ventral rami)
Head and Neck	
Scalenes (anterior, middle)	C4-C6 (anterior), ventral rami of cervical spinal nerves (middle)
Longus capitis	C1-C3 spinal nerves (ventral rami)
Longus colli	C2-C6 spinal nerves (ventral rami)
Rectus capitis anterior	C1-C2 spinal nerve branches

Moving AnatoME Exercise

Back, Neck, and Head Flexion: Pilates Roll Up

See Fig. 6.8 and Video 6.1.

- Starting position: Lying supine on the floor. Legs are extended and adducted (or hip distance apart). Shoulders are flexed with arms overhead, fingertips reaching behind you.
- Inhale and flex the shoulders to 90 degrees, bringing the fingertips toward the ceiling. Then, nod your chin to initiate flexion in the cervical spine.
- Exhale and engage the abdominals to flex the spine, sequentially articulating the cervical, thoracic, and lumbar vertebrae off of the mat, as if you could move them one by one. Keep the spine flexed and feet dorsiflexed as you roll up and over an imaginary ball, using the strength of your abdominals and the flexibility of your spine (not momentum) to enable this motion; if you need additional assistance to roll up, bend your knees and hold gently behind your thighs. Continue rolling until you are in a seated position with the spine flexed, arms reaching toward the feet parallel to the ground, cervical spine neutral with your gaze toward your knees.
- Inhale and draw the navel in toward the spine, using the lower abdominals to initiate the roll back toward the floor; sequentially articulate through the lumbar, thoracic, and cervical vertebrae, one by one.
- Exhale and continue flexing the shoulders to reach the fingertips behind you.
- Repeat five to six times.
- Ending position: Remain supine and relax your arms by your sides.

CLINICAL FOCUS 6.2   **Spinal Stenosis**

Spinal stenosis is a prevalent cause of chronic neck and lower back pain in the older adult population. It refers to a narrowing of the spinal canal and/or intervertebral foramina. Such stenoses are typically due to degenerative changes of the vertebral column that can result in a compression of the spinal cord or nerves. Stenoses can occur at single or multiple levels, with the lumbar and cervical spines most commonly affected because they are the most mobile and subject to wear and tear. Developing over a period of years, symptoms begin to appear around the sixth decade of life and commonly include pain and neuropathic symptoms such as weakness and numbness; the classic presentation of lumbar stenosis is unilateral

or bilateral radiating leg pain provoked by walking a short distance and relieved by rest and/or bending forward (as flexion opens the foramina, thereby alleviating symptoms). Although forward flexion of the spine is a preferred position for individuals affected with spinal stenosis, the spinal extensors should not be ignored. Strengthening these muscles not only helps stabilize the core but also helps promote a more neutral posture. Tailor extension exercises according to pain tolerance and ability. For example, modify the **Pilates Swimming** (see Video 13.3) exercise to lift only one arm or leg at a time; if lying prone is a problem, perform the exercise on hands and knees.

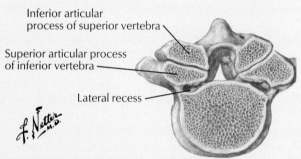

Inferior articular process of superior vertebra

Superior articular process of inferior vertebra

Lateral recess

Central spinal canal narrowed by enlargement of inferior articular process of superior vertebra. Lateral recesses narrowed by subluxation and osteophytic enlargement of superior articular processes of inferior vertebra.

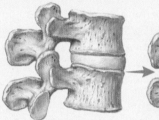
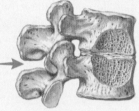

Properly spaced lumbar vertebrae with normal intervertebral disc

Vertebrae approximated due to loss of disc height. Subluxated articular process of inferior vertebra has encroached on foramen. Internal disruption of disc shown in cut section.

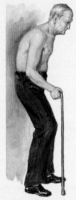

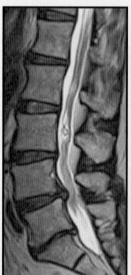
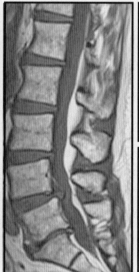
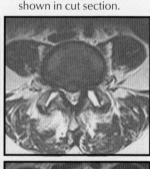

Patient assumes characteristic bent-over posture, with neck, spine, hips, and knees flexed; back is flat or convex, with absence of normal lordotic curvature. Pressure on cauda equina and resultant pain are thus relieved.

Combined spinal stenosis

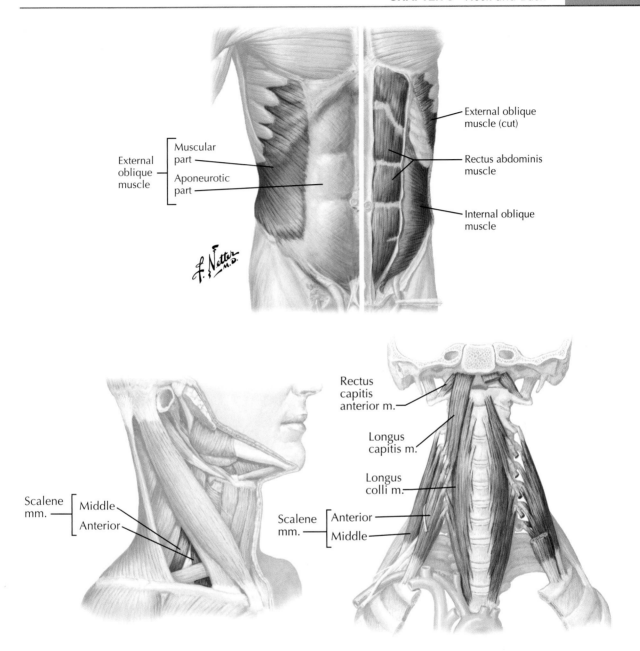

Fig. 6.7. Muscles that flex the vertebral column.

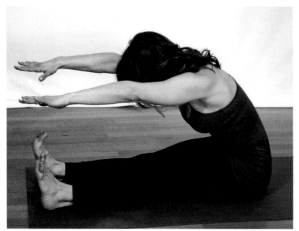

Fig. 6.8. Back, neck, and head flexion: **Pilates Roll Up** (see Video 6.1).

EXTENSION

Back Extension

Gymnasts engage in an impressive extension during a back walkover. Extension occurs as the reverse of flexion, bringing the posterior surfaces of two vertebrae closer together. It occurs as the inferior facets of a superior vertebra glide down and back along the superior facets of the vertebra below it; this allows the superior vertebral body to tilt posteriorly atop of the intervening intervertebral disc. As a whole, these actions compress the intervertebral disc posteriorly and expand it anteriorly. Limiting factors of extension include the tension provided by anterior spinal ligaments and the shape of the spinous processes. For example, thoracic extension is limited by the long, inferiorly sloping spinous processes of thoracic vertebrae, which can get in the way of one another (Clinical Focus 6.3 and see Practice What You Preach 6.1).

Head and Neck Extension

Many everyday movements, such as glancing up to check the weather, involve the combined actions of head and neck extension. The head moves at the atlantooccipital joint as the occipital condyles roll posteriorly upon the facets of the atlas. At the atlantoaxial joint, the atlas pivots backward upon the axis. In the lower intracervical articulations, extension occurs as the reverse of flexion; extension is initiated in the lower spine at C4-C7, with the inferior articular facets of the superior vertebrae sliding inferiorly and posteriorly, relative to the superior articular facets of the inferior vertebrae.

CLINICAL FOCUS 6.3
Nonspecific Back Pain

Chances are that you know someone who suffers from back pain. A daily reality for millions of Americans, lower back pain symptoms can be hard to pinpoint and difficult to describe. Some know it as back strain, back sprain, mechanical back pain, or lumbago, but these specific diagnoses are rarely made due to lack of a focal anatomical lesion. Hence, "nonspecific back pain" has become a catch-all term for general back complaints that escape a precise diagnosis. Although the typical onset follows some form of physical activity, such as lifting a heavy object, affected individuals may not recall exactly how or when the pain began. Symptoms, such as mild to moderate pain, occur most frequently in the lower back, the region of our vertebral column that carries the greatest load. Deconditioned core muscles (see Movement: The Core), which are epidemic in our computer-oriented society, also predispose an individual to muscle imbalances, lower back weakness, and possible injury. Take preventive steps and regularly strengthen the core muscles with exercises like the **Pilates Pelvic Tilts** (see Video 13.2) or the **Yoga Plank Pose** (see Video 8.4).

Try **Moving AnatoME** with **Yoga Cobra Pose** (Video 6.2) and lift your hands off the floor to notice the range of extension available when you engage only your spinal extensors (and not your arm muscles). Be mindful not to overcompensate for the limited range by hyperextending the neck.

Approximate Range of Motion

- Back: 40 degrees (thoracic = 25 degrees; lumbar = 15 degrees)
- Head and neck: 85 degrees

Muscles and Innervation

See Fig. 6.9.

Muscle	Nerve
Back	
Erector spinae (lower divisions)	Spinal nerves (dorsal rami)
Transversospinales (lower divisions)	Spinal nerves (dorsal rami)
Quadratus lumborum	T12-L4 (ventral rami)
Interspinales (lower divisions)	Spinal nerves (dorsal rami)

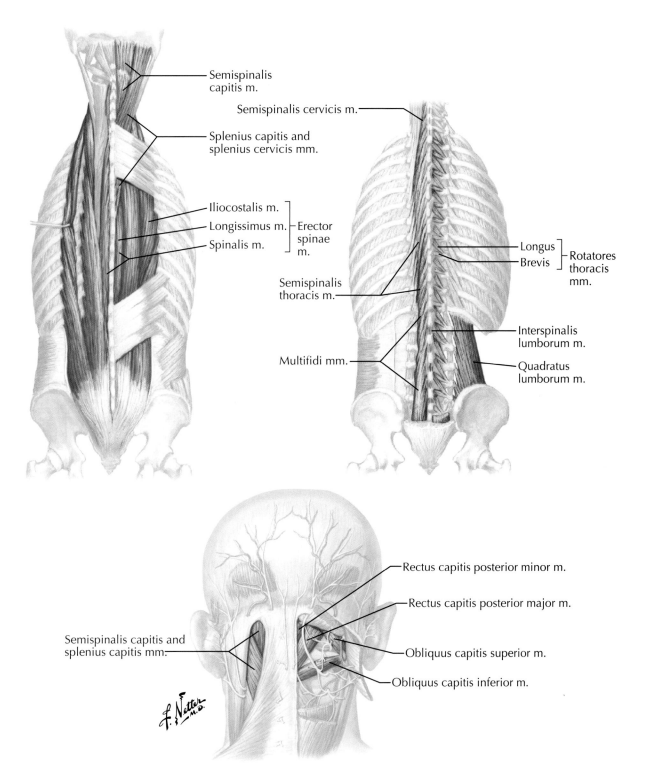

Semispinalis capitis m.

Semispinalis cervicis m.

Splenius capitis and splenius cervicis mm.

Iliocostalis m.
Longissimus m. — Erector spinae m.
Spinalis m.

Semispinalis thoracis m.

Multifidi mm.

Longus
Brevis — Rotatores thoracis mm.

Interspinalis lumborum m.

Quadratus lumborum m.

Rectus capitis posterior minor m.

Rectus capitis posterior major m.

Semispinalis capitis and splenius capitis mm.

Obliquus capitis superior m.

Obliquus capitis inferior m.

Fig. 6.9. Muscles that extend the vertebral column. (*Muscle not shown:* trapezius.)

Muscle	Nerve
Head and Neck	
Splenius capitis	Middle cervical nerves (dorsal rami)
Splenius cervicis	Middle cervical nerves (dorsal rami)
Erector spinae (superior divisions)	Spinal nerves (dorsal rami)
Transversospinales (superior divisions)	Spinal nerves (dorsal rami)
Interspinales (superior divisions)	Spinal nerves (dorsal rami)
Trapezius (upper fibers)	Accessory nerve (cranial nerve XI) and C2-C4
Rectus capitis posterior major and minor	Suboccipital nerve (C1)
Obliquus capitis superior and inferior	Suboccipital nerve (C1)

Moving AnatoME Exercise
Back, Neck, and Head Extension:
Yoga Cobra Pose (Bhujangasana)

▶ See Fig. 6.10 and Video 6.2.

- Starting position: Lying prone on the floor. Hands are flat on the floor, directly under your shoulders; fingers are spread, elbows bent, and arms adducted. Legs are elongated and hip distance apart, with the tops of your feet pressed into the floor.
- Inhale and begin to extend your elbows, extending your spine to lift your chest off the floor. The lift should arise from the strength of your back, not your

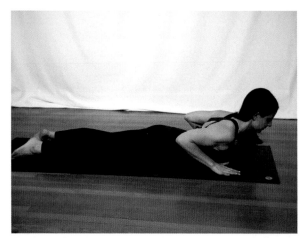

Fig. 6.10. Back, neck, and head extension: **Yoga Cobra Pose (Bhujangasana)** (see Video 6.2).

arms. Hips and legs stay on the ground; legs are active but buttocks are not gripped.

- Extend your elbows only to the height at which you can maintain a connection between your pubic bone and the floor, which might mean that your elbows remain flexed. Keep your shoulders depressed and away from your ears.
- Make sure that your head and neck are aligned as a continuation of the rest of your spine and are not hyperextended or hyperflexed; your gaze should fall diagonally on the floor in front of you.
- Maintain the pose for five rounds of breath.
- Ending position: Exhale and slowly release your torso to the floor.

LATERAL FLEXION
Back Lateral Flexion

Tilt your torso to one side as if you were carrying a heavy bag; this movement demonstrates lateral flexion, a side-bending of the spine. Like its forward counterpart, lateral flexion decreases the space between two vertebral bodies, but on their sides, as opposed to their anterior surfaces. Think about *left* lateral flexion to demonstrate how it occurs: the left sides of two adjacent vertebral bodies hinge together as their left superior and inferior facets glide together and their right facets glide apart; this action compresses the intervertebral disc on the left and expands it on the right. Often, this movement is believed to be coupled with slight vertebral rotation. Limiting factors include tension provided by contralateral spinal ligaments and muscles, as well as the presence of the rib cage.

Head and Neck Lateral Flexion

Huh? You perform some degree of head and neck lateral flexion, a movement that brings your ear closer to your shoulder, every day to convey sentiments such as curiosity or confusion. Like lateral flexion of the back, lateral flexion of the head and neck decreases the space between the lateral aspects of two vertebral bodies. This movement occurs to a minimal degree at the atlantooccipital joint, but most of it happens in the rest of the cervical spine (C2-C7), via the same mechanics described above.

Try **Moving AnatoME** with **Yoga Extended Side Angle Pose** (Video 6.3). Notice how lateral flexors on the ▶ ipsilateral side contract to get you into the pose, and your contralateral lateral flexors fire isometrically to prevent your torso from giving in to the force of gravity.

Approximate Range of Motion

- Back: 45 degrees in each direction (thoracic = 25 degrees; lumbar = 20 degrees)
- Head and neck: 40 degrees

Muscles and Innervation

See Fig. 6.11.

Muscle	Nerve
Back	
Erector spinae (lower divisions)	Spinal nerves (dorsal rami)
External oblique	T6-T12 (ventral rami) and subcostal nerve
Internal oblique	T6-L1 (ventral rami)
Quadratus lumborum	T12-L4 (ventral rami)
Transversospinales (lower divisions)	Spinal nerves (dorsal rami)
Psoas major	L1-L4
Intertransversarii (lower divisions)	Spinal nerves (dorsal and ventral rami)
Head and Neck	
Trapezius (upper fibers)	Accessory nerve (cranial nerve XI) and C2-C4
Sternocleidomastoid	Spinal root of accessory nerve (cranial nerve XI)
Scalenes	C3-C8
Splenius capitis	Middle cervical nerves (dorsal rami)
Splenius cervicis	Middle cervical nerves (dorsal rami)
Longus capitis	C1-C3 spinal nerves (ventral rami)
Longus colli	C2-C6 spinal nerves (ventral rami)
Erector spinae (superior divisions)	Spinal nerves (dorsal rami)
Obliquus capitis superior	Suboccipital nerve (C1)
Rectus capitis anterior	C1-C2 spinal nerve branches
Rectus capitis lateralis	C1-C2 spinal nerve branches
Rectus capitis posterior major and minor	Suboccipital nerve (C1)
Transversospinales (superior divisions)	Spinal nerves (dorsal rami)
Intertransversarii (superior divisions)	Spinal nerves (dorsal rami)

Moving AnatoME Exercise

Back, Head, and Neck Lateral Flexion:

Yoga Extended Side Angle Pose
(Utthita Parsvakonasana)

See Fig. 6.12 and Video 6.3.

- Starting position: Standing with your feet hip distance apart, in their natural parallel position. Weight is centered between both feet. Arms relax by your sides.
- Abduct your arms to 90 degrees, and step your feet apart so that your ankles align under your wrists. Keep your shoulders down, wrists neutral, and fingers elongated.
- Turn your left foot slightly inward (15 to 45 degrees) and your right foot 90 degrees outward. Align your left and right heels.
- Flex your right knee to 90 degrees, so that your thigh parallels the floor (or as close to parallel as possible). Position your knee directly over your ankle, in line with your second toe. Your entire foot should be flat on the floor with the arch engaged (no portion of your heel or toes should be lifted); all points of your left foot should equally touch the ground, as well.
- Exhale and laterally flex the spine, bending the right side of your torso toward your right thigh. Simultaneously, further abduct your left arm, raising it toward your head with your left palm facing toward the floor. Your right forearm rests on your right thigh; actively push the forearm and thigh against each other.
- On an inhale, stretch from the outside of your left foot through your left fingertips, lengthening the entire left side of your body; depress your scapula so there is space between your left shoulder and ear. Likewise, create length along your right side.
- Rotate your head to look at your left arm (otherwise, keep your head neutral).
- Stay in this position for five slow and deliberate breaths.
- Inhale and lift your torso to a neutral position, while bringing both arms back to 90 degrees. Extend your right knee, and return your feet to parallel.
- Reverse directions and repeat to the left side.
- Ending position: Relax your arms and return your feet to a hip distance stance.

ROTATION

Kayakers rotate their spines in order to place their paddles in the water and propel their boats forward. In the body, rotation is defined as movement of a part

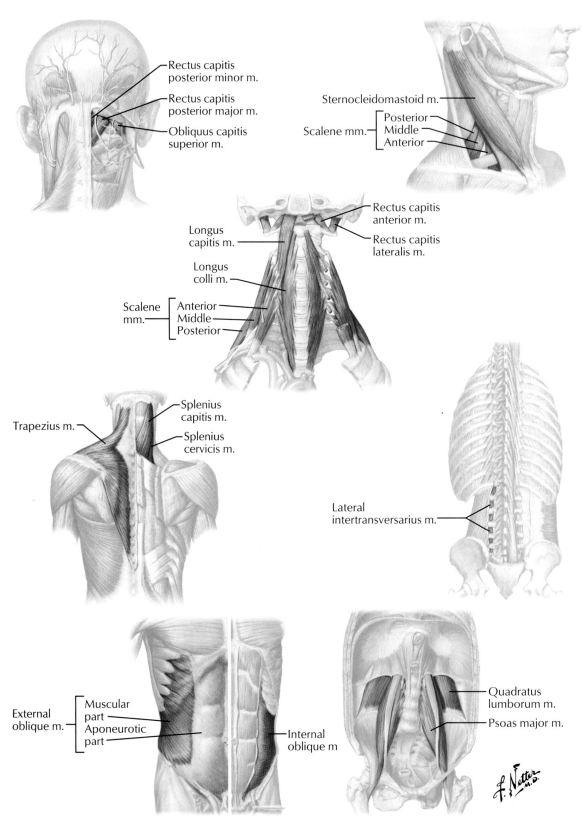

Fig. 6.11. Muscles that laterally flex the vertebral column. (*Muscles not shown:* erector spinae, transversospinales.)

Labels within the figure:

- Rectus capitis posterior minor m.
- Rectus capitis posterior major m.
- Obliquus capitis superior m.
- Sternocleidomastoid m.
- Scalene mm. — Posterior / Middle / Anterior
- Longus capitis m.
- Rectus capitis anterior m.
- Rectus capitis lateralis m.
- Longus colli m.
- Scalene mm. — Anterior / Middle / Posterior
- Trapezius m.
- Splenius capitis m.
- Splenius cervicis m.
- Lateral intertransversarius m.
- External oblique m. — Muscular part / Aponeurotic part
- Internal oblique m.
- Quadratus lumborum m.
- Psoas major m.

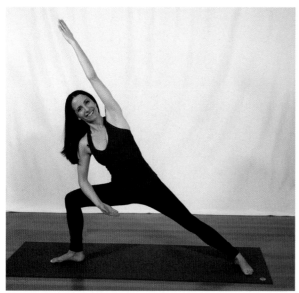

Fig. 6.12. Back, head, and neck lateral flexion: **Yoga Extended Side Angle Pose (Utthita Parsvakonasana)** (see Video 6.3).

around an axis; because the spine's vertical axis is the midline of the body, there is no "internal" or "external" rotation. Rotation of the spine, therefore, rotates the back to the left or right. At an invertebral level, rotation occurs as inferior articular facets of a vertebra above slide against the superior articular facets of the vertebra below. As a whole, this enables the superior vertebra to rotate atop of an intervertebral disc; a small amount of ipsilateral side-bending occurs concurrently. The orientation of facets primarily determines the degree of rotation allowed in different spinal segments. For instance, the lumbar region exhibits very little range owing to its vertically oriented facets, which collide with one another during rotation. The cervical and upper thoracic regions, with more horizontally aligned facets, are able to rotate the most.

Head and Neck Rotation

No, nope, no way. There may be different ways of disagreeing, but everyone performs disapproving gestures in the same way: with head and neck rotation. Nearly half of head rotation occurs at the atlantoaxial joint, as the atlas pivots about the dens of the axis. The head rotates in conjunction with the atlas, as one unit relative to the axis. Rotation continues throughout the rest of the cervical

spine guided by the oblique orientation of the facet joints, and via similar mechanisms as described above (Practice What You Preach 6.2).

Try **Moving AnatoME** with **Pilates Spine Twist** (Video 6.4) and experience how each segment of the spine exhibits specific ranges of movement, with your cervical spine having the most. Although this innate flexibility exists, keep your cervical spine in line with the rest of your vertebral column during the exercise.

Approximate Range of Motion

- Back: 35 degrees in each direction (thoracic = 30 degrees; lumbar = 5 degrees)
- Head and neck: 90 degrees in each direction; 180 degrees of total rotational motion. Of note, with the addition of about 150 degrees of total horizontal plane motion of the eyes, the visual field approaches 360 degrees without moving the trunk.

Muscles and Innervation

See Fig. 6.13.

Muscle	Nerve
Back	
External oblique	T6-T12 (ventral rami) and subcostal nerve
Internal oblique	T6-L1 (ventral rami)
Transversospinales	Spinal nerves (dorsal rami)
Erector spinae	Spinal nerves (dorsal rami)
Head and Neck	
Sternocleidomastoid	Spinal root of accessory nerve (cranial nerve XI)
Splenius capitis	Middle cervical nerves (dorsal rami)
Splenius cervicis	Middle cervical nerves (dorsal rami)
Rectus capitis posterior major	Suboccipital nerve (C1)
Obliquus capitis inferior	Suboccipital nerve (C1)
Trapezius (upper fibers)	Accessory nerve (cranial nerve XI) and C2-C4
Erector spinae (superior divisions)	Spinal nerves (dorsal rami)
Transversospinales (superior divisions)	Spinal nerves (dorsal rami)
Scalene (anterior)	C4-6

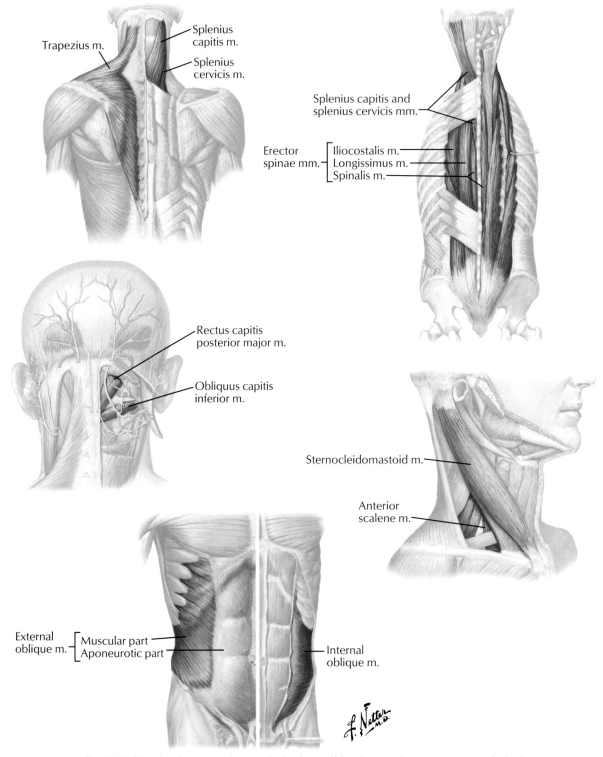

Fig. 6.13. Muscles that rotate the vertebral column. (*Muscles not shown:* transversospinales.)

Your neck is, and should be operated as, a natural extension of your spine, as in the **Yoga Cobra Pose** (see Video 6.2). Sometimes, however, its connection to your torso feels stiff and tense as your shoulders creep closer to your ears (see Practice What You Preach 8.2). Keep this region mobile by doing head and neck circles. Start by rolling your head slowly to the front, side, back, side, and front. Keep your torso still and shoulders relaxed. Perform the circles as if you had a small ball between your head and neck (this will prevent you from moving your head through an excessive range of motion). Repeat five times, ending with your head in its neutral position before you reverse directions. To add an extra measure of relaxation, close your eyes and add breath: Every time your head extends, take a slow, deep inhale; when your head flexes, enjoy a slow, deep exhale.

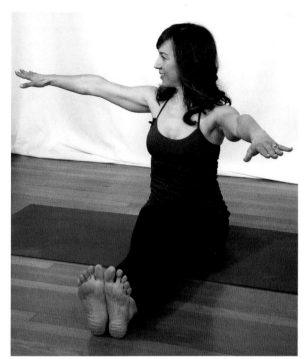

Fig. 6.14. Back, head, and neck rotation: **Pilates Spine Twist** (see Video 6.4).

Moving AnatoME Exercise
Back, Head, and Neck Rotation: Pilates Spine Twist

See Fig. 6.14 and Video 6.4.

- Starting position: Sitting on the floor with legs extended and adducted in front of you, ankles dorsiflexed (sit on a cushion or atop of a rolled-up edge of your mat if you need help sitting erect atop of your sitting bones). Bring your arms in a wide V in front of you, parallel to the ground with palms facing down. Maintain this arm position throughout the exercise.
- Inhale to prepare, and lengthen from your pelvis to the crown of your head.
- Exhale and rotate the spine to the right. Make sure to keep your pelvis neutral with the left sitting bone on the mat.
- Inhale and unwind slightly to the left.
- Exhale and rotate further to the right.
- Inhale and unwind slightly to the left.
- Exhale and rotate a little further to the right.
- Inhale and return to center.
- Repeat to the left side. Then repeat the full exercise four to six times.
- Ending position: Return to center and relax the arms by your sides.

MOVEMENT: THE CORE

In addition to moving the vertebral column, the abdominal muscles play an important role as part of the core. The core is a network of muscles that stabilize the spine and enable proper posture in all activities—whether you are sitting, standing, swimming, or skiing. The concept of the core has been around for a long time but became popularized in the 1990s, when research in Australian physiotherapy laboratories demonstrated a correlation between the timing of the activation of trunk muscles and the development of back injury and lower back pain. The core has since gained prominence in physiatry offices and Pilates studios alike as a way of referring to an area of the body that, when strengthened, can help maintain ideal alignment and also prevent lower back injury. Despite its popularity, however, not much is scientifically known about the core, because it is not a concretely defined region of the body; indeed, many different interpretations exist as to its constituent parts. Most interpretations include some or all of the following (Fig. 6.15):

- **The "roof":** the diaphragm
- **The "floor":** the pelvic diaphragm muscles

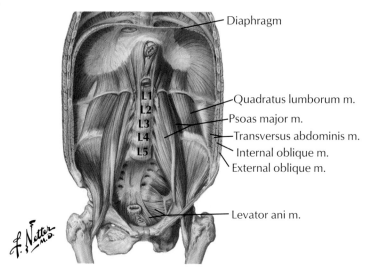

Fig. 6.15. Examples of muscles classified as part of the core.

- **Posterior supports:** the transversospinales muscles (notably the multifidus muscle) and erector spinae muscles
- **Anterolateral supports:** all four anterior abdominal wall muscles, notably the transversus abdominis muscle (Clinical Focus 6.4)
- **Frequently included structures:** the quadratus lumborum, psoas major, intertransversarii, and interspinales muscles

What is known about the core is that the term refers, generally, to anatomically and functionally interconnected muscles of the lower back, abdomen, and pelvis, which function synergistically to stabilize the spine. Spinal stability is important because it allows the trunk to maintain a static (and, hence, protective) posture, even in the face of destabilizing external forces; these forces may come from any place external to the trunk, whether it is a slanted floor, a moving subway, a person who is pushing you, or the movements of your arms and legs. Additionally, limbs function more efficiently when the trunk is stable. Imagine, for example, holding a 50-pound box without a strong trunk. The box's weight would then be supported mainly by your two upper extremities, which (1) would not likely be strong enough to bear the full burden and (2) would end up suffering strain or, worse, dislocation.

Stabilization by a core set of muscles does not imply, however, that the human body has only one, designated set of stabilization muscles; core muscles work synergistically

CLINICAL FOCUS 6.4
Abdominal Hernia

A herniation is an abnormal protrusion of contents from one space into another. In the abdomen, a hernia refers to a protrusion of a peritoneal sac with or without abdominal contents therein. Many different types of hernias can occur, including inguinal, femoral, and umbilical. Inguinal hernias occur most commonly, especially in men. They occur in the inguinal region, located at the junction between the anterior abdominal wall and the thigh, an area otherwise known as the groin. In this region, the abdominal wall is intrinsically weak from changes during embryonic development; a peritoneal sac can thus protrude through the weak area in the wall, creating an inguinal hernia that potentially protrudes all the way into a man's scrotum, or into a woman's labia majus. An increase in abdominal pressure is the primary cause of protrusion, precipitated by a chronic cough, heavy lifting, or abdominal wall muscle deconditioning. Strengthening the muscles of the abdominal wall is important in preventing the development or worsening of an abdominal hernia. Remember, however, that many exercises that strengthen the abdominal muscles also increase intraabdominal pressure; this is a catch-22 situation with hernias. Choose exercises, accordingly, that engage the transversus abdominis muscle (eg, **Pilates Pelvic Tilts**, Video 13.2); exercises such as the **Yoga Malasana Pose** (a deep squat) would not be recommended.

with many others to accomplish that task. What, then, distinguishes the core muscles? In addition to their purpose, they are distinguished (1) by their location, forming an enclosed core-set around the trunk of the body, and (2) by their subsequent encompassing of the body's center of mass, which is located in the midline of the body, anterior to the second sacral vertebra (approximately at the level of the posterior superior iliac spines). The center of mass is important because the rest of the body (or the rest of the mass of any system, for that matter) behaves as if all of its mass were concentrated there; as a result, the center of mass is the point around which the body can be balanced. For instance, when standing on one leg in the **Yoga Tree Pose** (see Video 13.1), once you find your center, it does not matter how your free leg is positioned (whether your foot is resting on your ankle versus your calf versus your inner thigh); your balance will not be disturbed. It will likewise not be disturbed if your hands are in the prayer position in front of your heart or above you, reaching toward the sky. But the converse is also true: If you are unable to find your center, you will have difficulty standing on one leg, regardless of where the free foot is placed.

The core, therefore, may not only play a role in spinal stabilization, but it may also be a poignant reminder of the importance of proprioception during activity and of further proprioceptive principles, such as stabilization, center of mass, and balance, which can be applied to all activities (Practice What You Preach 6.3).

Moving AnatoME

With every step you take and every exercise in this book, you can and should engage your core muscles. To hone in on some of them, try exercises such as the **Yoga Cobra Pose** (see Video 6.2), **Yoga Plank Pose** (see Video 8.4),

Pilates Pelvic Tilts (see Video 13.2), **Pilates Spine Twist** (see Video 6.4), and **Pilates Leg Pull Prep** (see Video 10.2).

MOVEMENT: RESPIRATION

Respiration involves the exchange of gases (oxygen and carbon dioxide) between the atmosphere and the body's cells; ventilation is the mechanical process by which breathing occurs. You respire (breathe) to create energy. Each time you inhale, you consume oxygen provided by the environment (eg, trees, plants) to generate a type of energy called adenosine triphosphate (ATP) during cellular respiration. ATP is the energy currency of your body; it fuels every cell, allowing you to walk, run, breathe, and live. Exhalation, conversely, returns carbon dioxide to the environment, for use there as energy (ie, trees photosynthesize carbon dioxide into sugars, food).

Nearly all of the time, inhalation and exhalation occur involuntarily, guided by the autonomic nervous system. When commands from the cerebral cortex of the brain override the brainstem, however, breathing becomes voluntary, for instance, when you take a large gulp of air before diving underwater. Breathing is therefore one of the few physiologic processes that can be both involuntary and voluntary.

Inhalation

The primary muscle of respiration is the diaphragm. At rest, this muscle naturally domes upward into the chest. To inspire air, the muscle contracts, flattening its shape and pushing down upon the abdominal contents. Assisting the diaphragm during inspiration are the external intercostals (among other muscles), which take part by lifting the ribs up and out. This "bucket-handle" mechanism of elevation occurs as the neck of a rib moves around an axis of rotation between the costotransverse and costovertebral joints; a subsequent torsion occurs at the sternocostal joint. These combined movements result in a vertical, anteroposterior, and lateral expansion of the thoracic cavity, a change in shape that also increases the intrathoracic volume. As the volume of the cavity increases, the pressure of the cavity decreases, initiating a flow of air into the lungs. If a more vigorous inspiration is needed (eg, during exercise), the body enlists secondary and accessory respiratory muscles to expand the rib cage at a more rapid rate (eg, scalene muscles). This process helps the body supply more oxygen to tissues during times of increased demand.

PRACTICE WHAT YOU PREACH 6.3
The Core of the Matter

Carve out 5 minutes every day to get to the core of the matter: in this case, yours. First, engage the abdominal muscles and pelvic diaphragm with the **Pilates Pelvic Tilts** (see Video 13.2), and then roll over to strengthen your lower back muscles with the **Yoga Cobra Pose** (see Video 6.2). You will stand straighter, move more efficiently, and be glad that you supported yourself so that you can better support others.

Exhalation

Exhalation is the reverse process of inhalation, with the diaphragm relaxing; its dome recoils upward into its resting position. The rib cage likewise recoils as the other muscles of inhalation also relax, and the internal and innermost intercostals may help depress the ribs. These combined movements allow the ribs to return to their resting position, thereby decreasing the intrathoracic volume. The decreased volume results in increased pressure, so air moves from the higher-pressure state of the lungs to the lower-pressure state of the atmosphere. Quiet expiration is primarily a passive process that does not depend on muscle activation. During exercise, when there is an increased need to release carbon dioxide back into the atmosphere (following an increased intake of oxygen), the secondary and accessory muscles may assist. For instance, contraction of the abdominal muscles actively compresses the thoracic cavity, pushing up the diaphragm and forcefully expelling air.

Rest

Between each exhalation and inhalation is a period when the pressure gradient between the atmosphere and alveoli is zero. The diaphragm thus remains at equilibrium, with no air moving into or out of the lungs (Box 6.4).

Muscles of Respiration

See Fig. 6.16.

Muscle	Inhalation	Exhalation
Primary	Diaphragm	Diaphragm
Secondary	External intercostals	Internal and innermost intercostals
	Serratus posterior superior and inferior	Transversus thoracis
	Levatores costarum	Subcostals

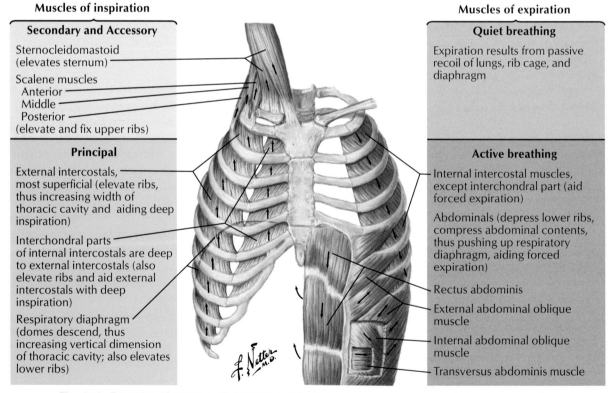

Muscles of inspiration

Secondary and Accessory

Sternocleidomastoid (elevates sternum)

Scalene muscles
Anterior
Middle
Posterior
(elevate and fix upper ribs)

Principal

External intercostals, most superficial (elevate ribs, thus increasing width of thoracic cavity and aiding deep inspiration)

Interchondral parts of internal intercostals are deep to external intercostals (also elevate ribs and aid external intercostals with deep inspiration)

Respiratory diaphragm (domes descend, thus increasing vertical dimension of thoracic cavity; also elevates lower ribs)

Muscles of expiration

Quiet breathing

Expiration results from passive recoil of lungs, rib cage, and diaphragm

Active breathing

Internal intercostal muscles, except interchondral part (aid forced expiration)

Abdominals (depress lower ribs, compress abdominal contents, thus pushing up respiratory diaphragm, aiding forced expiration)

Rectus abdominis

External abdominal oblique muscle

Internal abdominal oblique muscle

Transversus abdominis muscle

Fig. 6.16. Examples of muscles of respiration. (*Muscles not shown:* serratus posterior, levator costae, pectoralis minor, transversus thoracis.)

BOX 6.4	**A Better Breath**

Perhaps you have heard references made to abdominal (belly) breaths and thoracic (chest) breaths. What is the difference? When one takes an abdominal breath, one actively engages the diaphragm during ventilation. As the muscle flattens during inspiration, the pressure within the abdominal cavity increases, causing a protrusion of the abdomen; during exhalation, the abdominal muscles contract to help expel air as the diaphragm relaxes, causing the abdomen to recoil. These in-and-out abdominal movements are the cardinal signs of well-done abdominal breathing, which richly perfuses the lungs with oxygen; it is important to use all of the lungs, since the bases, for example, are the most blood-rich areas (due to gravity). Overall, therefore, abdominal breathing is a physically—and some would say emotionally and spiritually—fulfilling way to breathe. Thoracic breathing, on the other hand, is a more shallow form of ventilation. Alone, this type of breath does not perfuse as much of the lungs.

A deeper breath results in greater gas exchange and nourishment for the body. Therefore, if you are unaware of your breath unintentionally stifling it in the upper thorax, you may be short-changing your body. Instead, breathe with both a belly and a chest breath for greatest effect.

Muscle	Inhalation	Exhalation
Accessory *(engaged in forceful inhalations/ exhalations)*	Serratus anterior	Transversus abdominis
	Sternocleidomastoid	Internal obliques
	Scalene muscles	External obliques
	Pectoralis major	Rectus abdominis
	Pectoralis minor	
	Trapezius	

Of note, the body has several strategies available for activating its respiratory muscles, depending on its workload. Despite extensive electromyographic studies, therefore, the precise respiratory roles of the individual intercostal muscles—along with the myriad secondary and accessory muscles—are difficult to interpret. In fact, any muscle that causes a shape change of the thoracoabdominal wall may be considered a respiratory muscle. Additionally, some anatomists believe that any muscle that is involved in contracting or expanding an orifice to allow air to enter or exit the body may be considered a muscle of respiration, which would even include the orbicularis oris muscle of the lips.

Try **Moving AnatoME** with **Alternate Nostril Breath (Anuloma Viloma)** (see Fig. 18.5 and Video 18.5).

Regional Overview of Upper Extremity

Beginning in the midline of the body and extending to the far reaches of the fingers, the upper extremity is an anatomical marvel. It allows for an expansive range of motion and accurate positioning of the hands in space, two features distinguishing humans and their primate relatives from the rest of the mammalian pack. Remember, not every creature can swing from a tree, hold a hammer, and write a list.

Each upper extremity is divided into discrete regions (Fig. 7.1):

- The **shoulder** is the area of the upper limb's attachment to the trunk. Although often thought of as one joint, the shoulder is actually a complex of several joints.
- The **arm** consists of the portion of the upper limb between the shoulder and the elbow.
- The **forearm** is the portion of the upper limb between the elbow and the wrist.
- The **hand** is the portion of the upper limb that is distal to the wrist.

BONES OF THE UPPER EXTREMITY

The skeletal framework of the upper extremity enables expansive reach and dexterity, and includes the following bones (Fig. 7.2):

- **Shoulder girdle:** Clavicle, scapula
- **Arm:** Humerus
- **Forearm:** Ulna, radius

- **Hand:**
  - **Carpal bones (lateral to medial):** Proximal row: scaphoid, lunate, triquetrum, pisiform; distal row: trapezium, trapezoid, capitate, hamate
  - **Metacarpal bones:** Metacarpals I, II, III, IV, V (lateral to medial)
  - **Phalanges (lateral to medial):** Proximal (fingers I to V), middle (fingers II to V), distal (fingers I to V)

MUSCLES OF THE UPPER EXTREMITY

The muscles responsible for moving these bones can be categorized regionally: scapulohumeral, thoracoappendicular, arm, forearm, and intrinsic hand muscles (Table 7.1 and Figs. 7.3, 7.4, and 7.5). For example, the supraspinatus, which abducts the arm, arises from the scapula and attaches to the humerus, hence, its classification as scapulohumeral.

The upper extremity muscles work harmoniously to bring about the major function of the entire extremity: positioning the hand in space to facilitate its work (eg, sensing, gripping, and manipulating objects). Why are all of these muscles needed for just a few hand movements? Recall that intricate hand motions are required to acquire food, make tools, and light fires, the very activities underlying our evolutionary ascent, continuation, and distinction from other species.

Anterior view

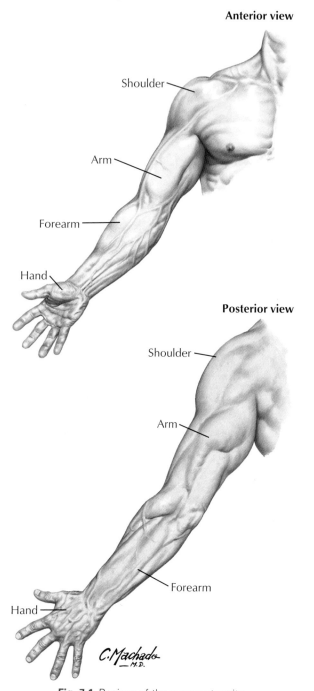

Shoulder

Arm

Forearm

Hand

Posterior view

Shoulder

Arm

Forearm

Hand

Fig. 7.1 Regions of the upper extremity.

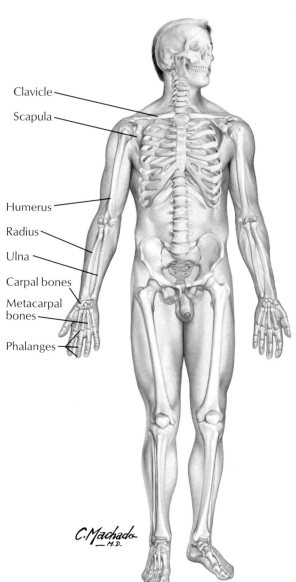

Clavicle

Scapula

Humerus

Radius

Ulna

Carpal bones

Metacarpal bones

Phalanges

Fig. 7.2 Bones of the upper extremity.

TABLE 7.1	**Muscle Groups of the Upper Extremity**	
Group	**Muscles**	**Notes**
Scapulohumeral	Deltoid, rotator cuff (supraspinatus, infraspinatus, teres minor, subscapularis), teres major	The scapulohumeral muscles link the scapula and the humerus, permitting each arm movement.
Thoracoappendicular	**Anterior:** Pectoralis major, pectoralis minor, serratus anterior, subclavius **Posterior:** Trapezius, levator scapulae, latissimus dorsi, rhomboid major and minor	The thoracoappendicular muscles link the thorax to the appendicular skeleton. They move the arm via the glenohumeral joint and scapulothoracic pseudojoint.
Arm	**Anterior:** Biceps brachii, brachialis, coracobrachialis **Posterior:** Triceps brachii	The anterior compartment houses muscles that generally flex the arm or forearm, whereas the posterior compartment muscle—there is only one—extends the arm.
Forearm	**Anterior (superficial):** Palmaris longus, flexor carpi radialis, flexor carpi ulnaris, pronator teres, flexor digitorum superficialis **Anterior (deep):** Flexor digitorum profundus, flexor pollicis longus, pronator quadratus **Posterior (superficial):** Brachioradialis, extensor carpi radialis longus, extensor carpi radialis brevis, extensor carpi ulnaris, extensor digitorum, extensor digiti minimi, anconeus **Posterior (deep):** Supinator, abductor pollicis longus, extensor pollicis brevis, extensor pollicis longus, extensor indices	The forearm is packed with 20 muscles that cross the wrist and/or elbow joints. In general, the anterior group includes muscles that flex the wrist and fingers and pronate the forearm. The posterior group includes muscles that extend the wrist and fingers and supinate the forearm.
Intrinsic hand	**Anterior:** Palmar brevis, adductor pollicis, palmar interossei (four muscles), lumbricals (four muscles) **Anterior (thenar):** Opponens pollicis, abductor pollicis brevis, flexor pollicis brevis **Anterior (hypothenar):** Opponens digiti minimi, abductor digiti minimi, flexor digiti minimi brevis **Posterior:** Dorsal interossei (four muscles)	On the anterior surface, the thenar and hypothenar groups contain muscles acting upon the thumb and little finger, respectively. The posterior compartment has only one muscle. All of the intrinsic hand muscles work together to move the fingers.

A. Scapulohumeral and thoracoappendicular muscles

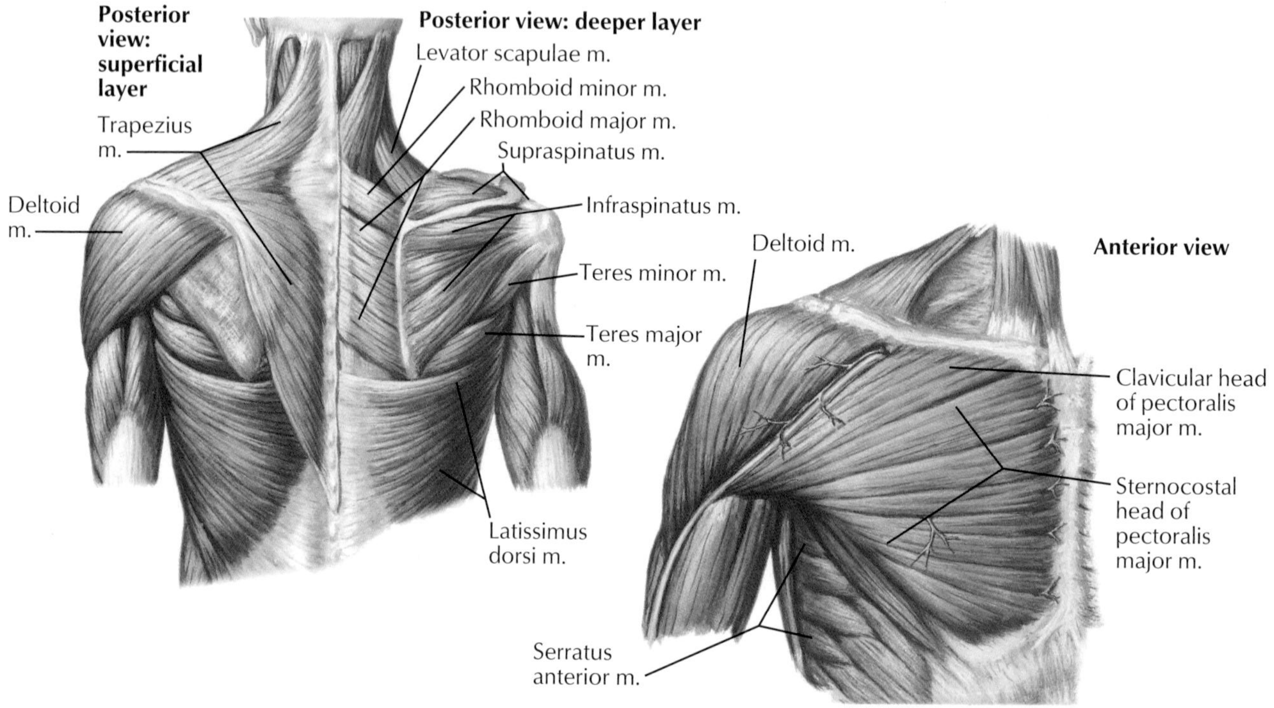

Posterior view: superficial layer

Trapezius m.

Deltoid m.

Posterior view: deeper layer

Levator scapulae m.

Rhomboid minor m.

Rhomboid major m.

Supraspinatus m.

Infraspinatus m.

Teres minor m.

Teres major m.

Latissimus dorsi m.

Deltoid m.

Anterior view

Clavicular head of pectoralis major m.

Sternocostal head of pectoralis major m.

Serratus anterior m.

B. Arm muscles

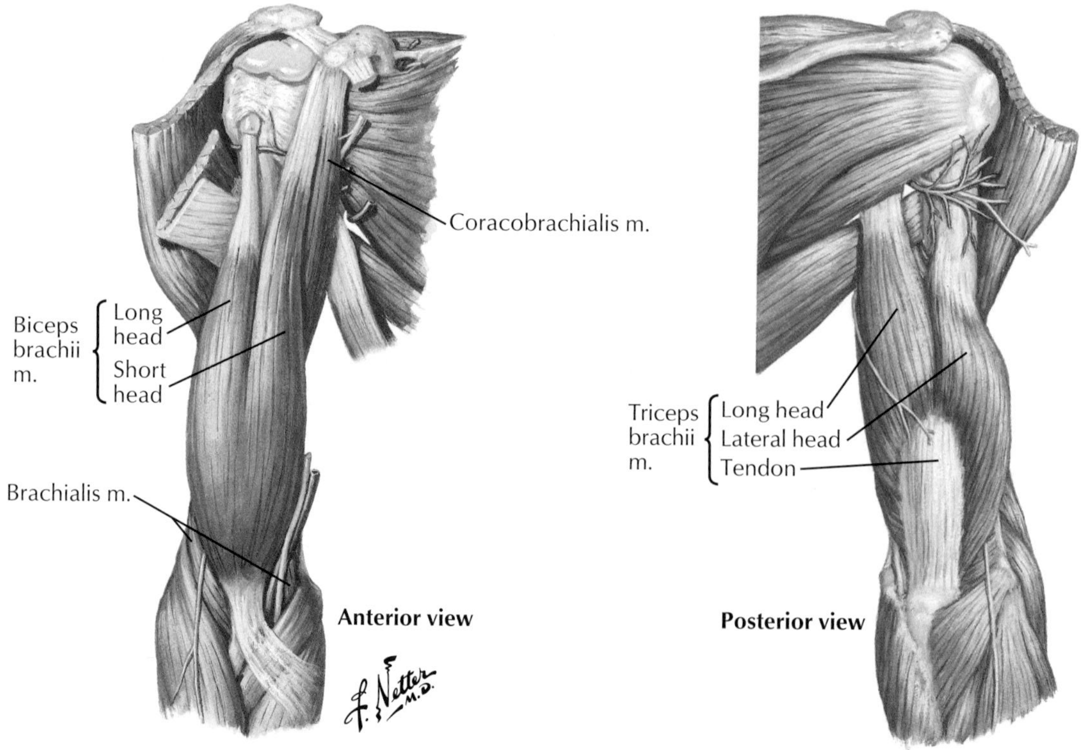

Coracobrachialis m.

Biceps brachii m.
- Long head
- Short head

Brachialis m.

Anterior view

Triceps brachii m.
- Long head
- Lateral head
- Tendon

Posterior view

f. Netter M.D.

Fig. 7.3 Scapulohumeral, thoracoappendicular, and arm muscles. *(Muscles not shown:* pectoralis minor, subscapularis, subclavius.)

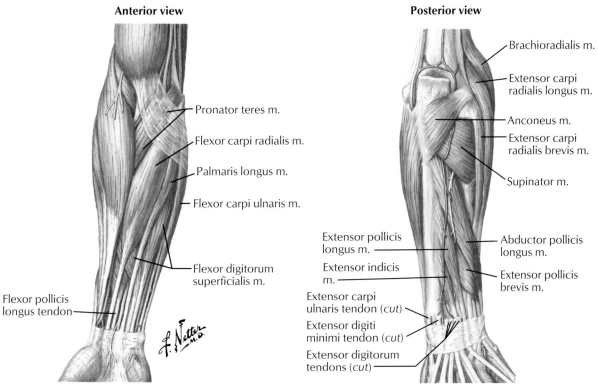

Anterior view

- Pronator teres m.
- Flexor carpi radialis m.
- Palmaris longus m.
- Flexor carpi ulnaris m.
- Flexor digitorum superficialis m.

Flexor pollicis longus tendon

f. Netter M.D.

Posterior view

- Brachioradialis m.
- Extensor carpi radialis longus m.
- Anconeus m.
- Extensor carpi radialis brevis m.
- Supinator m.
- Abductor pollicis longus m.
- Extensor pollicis brevis m.

Extensor pollicis longus m.

Extensor indicis m.

Extensor carpi ulnaris tendon (*cut*)

Extensor digiti minimi tendon (*cut*)

Extensor digitorum tendons (*cut*)

Fig. 7.4 Forearm muscles. *(Muscles not shown:* flexor digitorum profundus, flexor pollicis longus, pronator quadratus.)

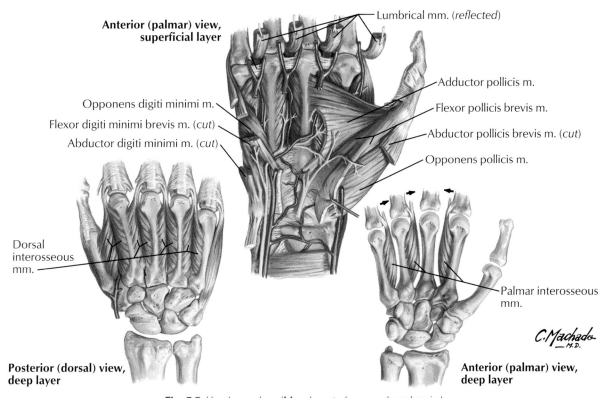

Anterior (palmar) view, superficial layer

Lumbrical mm. (*reflected*)

Opponens digiti minimi m.

Flexor digiti minimi brevis m. (*cut*)

Abductor digiti minimi m. (*cut*)

- Adductor pollicis m.
- Flexor pollicis brevis m.
- Abductor pollicis brevis m. (*cut*)
- Opponens pollicis m.

Dorsal interosseous mm.

Posterior (dorsal) view, deep layer

Palmar interosseous mm.

Anterior (palmar) view, deep layer

C. Machado M.D.

Fig. 7.5 Hand muscles. *(Muscle not shown:* palmar brevis.)

8

Shoulder

OVERVIEW

- The shoulder complex is formed by associated joints that connect the arm and axial skeleton.
- The articulations occur between the scapula and humerus (the glenohumeral joint), the scapula and clavicle (the acromioclavicular joint), the sternum and clavicle (the sternoclavicular joint), and the scapula and thorax (the scapulothoracic joint, which is a pseudojoint).
- Movements include:
  - **Arm:** Flexion, extension, abduction, adduction, external rotation, internal rotation, circumduction
  - **Scapula:** Elevation, depression, protraction, retraction, upward rotation, downward rotation
  - **Clavicle:** Elevation, depression, protraction, retraction, rotation
- Example exercises:
  - Elevation (**Pilates Scapula Isolations,** Video 8.1)
  - Depression (**Pilates Scapula Isolations,** Video 8.1)
  - Protraction (**Yoga Cat-Cow Pose,** Video 8.2)
  - Retraction (**Yoga Cat-Cow Pose,** Video 8.2)
  - Upward rotation (**Yoga Half Sun Salutation,** Video 8.3)
  - Downward rotation (**Yoga Half Sun Salutation,** Video 8.3)
  - Arm flexion (**Yoga Plank Pose,** Video 8.4)
  - Extension (**Yoga Upward Plank Pose,** Video 8.5)
  - Abduction (**Pilates Side Arm Series** [**Abduction/Adduction**]**,** Video 8.6)
  - Adduction (**Pilates Side Arm Series** [**Abduction/Adduction**]**,** Video 8.6)
  - External rotation (**Pilates Side Arm Series** [**Internal/External Rotation**]**,** Video 8.7)
  - Internal rotation (**Pilates Side Arm Series** [**Internal/External Rotation**]**,** Video 8.7)

STRUCTURE AND FUNCTION

Tap yourself on the shoulder. Thanks to the smooth curves of the deltoid muscle lying below the skin and above the acromion, the shoulder feels like one smooth region. Yet what most laypeople refer to simply as the shoulder is, anatomically, a complex of several joints made from several upper extremity structures. So what, exactly, is it?

The shoulder is the region of the upper limb's attachment to the trunk, composed of bones, muscles, joints, and other soft tissue structures. The clavicle and scapula together form the shoulder girdle (a.k.a. the pectoral girdle). The clavicle, scapula, and humerus, along with the joints they form with each other and with the axial skeleton, give rise to the shoulder complex. So while there is a "shoulder joint" (the glenohumeral joint), it is only one joint in a complex of four joints, which also includes the sternoclavicular, acromioclavicular, and scapulothoracic joints.

Each of these shoulder joints is functionally interdependent and vital to upper extremity movement. For example, if you raise your hand to ask a question in class, it may seem, at first glance, that you have used only your glenohumeral joint to flex your arm and accomplish this task. A closer look reveals an intricate employment of not only your glenohumeral joint but also your sternoclavicular, acromioclavicular, and scapulothoracic joints (Fig. 8.1). To fully grasp upper extremity movement, it is therefore important to understand the structure and function of each shoulder girdle joint as you keep the larger movement in mind.

Sternoclavicular Joint

The sternoclavicular (SC) joint is created by the medial end of the clavicle and the manubrium of the sternum, along with a small part of the costal cartilage of the first

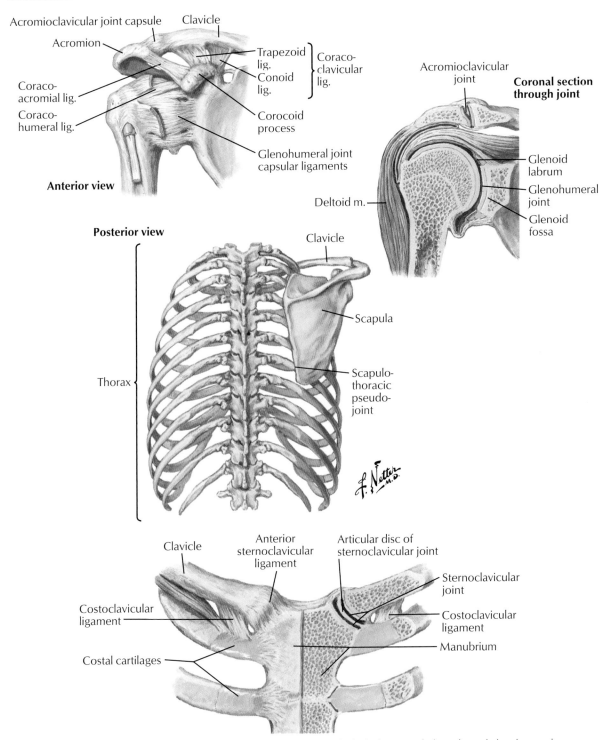

Acromioclavicular joint capsule

Clavicle

Acromion

Coraco-acromial lig.

Coraco-humeral lig.

Trapezoid lig.

Conoid lig.

Coraco-clavicular lig.

Corocoid process

Glenohumeral joint capsular ligaments

Anterior view

Acromioclavicular joint

Coronal section through joint

Glenoid labrum

Glenohumeral joint

Glenoid fossa

Deltoid m.

Posterior view

Clavicle

Scapula

Scapulo-thoracic pseudo-joint

Thorax

Clavicle

Anterior sternoclavicular ligament

Articular disc of sternoclavicular joint

Sternoclavicular joint

Costoclavicular ligament

Costoclavicular ligament

Costal cartilages

Manubrium

Fig. 8.1 Joints of the shoulder girdle (sternoclavicular, acromioclavicular, scapulothoracic, and glenohumeral joints).

rib (see Fig. 8.1). It is a saddle-shaped joint divided by an articular disc. Surrounded by a thick fibrous capsule and surrounding ligaments, the SC joint is incredibly strong—and for good reason, as it is the only bony attachment between the axial and upper appendicular skeletons. As a synovial joint, the SC joint also contributes to mobility. Although you may not notice its subtle movements, the SC joint allows small amounts of anteroposterior, vertical, and rotational motions of the clavicle, which affects mobility at the other shoulder complex joints.

Acromioclavicular Joint

The acromioclavicular (AC) joint is a small joint between the lateral end of the clavicle and the medial surface of the acromion (see Fig. 8.1). Like the SC joint, it is synovial and variably contains an articular disc. Unlike the strong SC joint, however, the AC joint is relatively weak and highly susceptible to injury (seen with shoulder separation, described in Clinical Focus 8.3). The strength it does have is imparted by intrinsic and accessory ligaments (eg, acromioclavicular, coracoacromial ligaments), as well as the muscular fibers of the trapezius, which helps fortify the joint superiorly. Like the SC joint, the AC joint functions as a "team player" in upper extremity movement. Microadjustments of the clavicle are enabled at the AC joint; they fine-tune articulations with the scapula and, by connection, the arm.

Scapulothoracic Joint

The term *scapulothoracic (ST) joint* is used to describe the relationship between the anterior surface of the scapula and the posterior thorax (see Fig. 8.1). It is technically not a true joint due to the absence of normal arthrologic structures such as capsules, cavities, and ligaments. However, it is classified as a false joint or pseudojoint due to (1) the interface between its two different bony surfaces and (2) its role in shoulder girdle movement. The movements of the scapula at the ST joint—elevation, depression, retraction, protraction, and upward and downward rotation—enable proper functioning of the glenohumeral joint and are, themselves, a result of individual motions of the SC and AC joints. It therefore interconnects the shoulder girdle joints and functions as a vital puzzle piece in upper extremity motion.

Glenohumeral (Shoulder) Joint

The "star" of the shoulder girdle is the glenohumeral (GH) joint (commonly considered *the* shoulder joint).

It is a synovial, ball-in-socket joint built to move, with a large ball, the head of the humerus, interfacing with a relatively small socket, the glenoid fossa of the scapula (Box 8.1). The unique shape of its articular surfaces permits a wealth of multiaxial movements: flexion, extension, abduction, adduction, and internal and external rotation, as well as circumduction. Both the humeral head and the glenoid fossa are covered with smooth hyaline cartilage, further assisting the joint's mobility. The joint itself is encased within a relatively loose fibrous capsule that attaches the rim of the glenoid fossa and the anatomical neck of the humerus. Like other synovial joints, the capsule's inner synovial membrane produces fluid, which nourishes the articular surfaces, decreases friction, and contributes to even more mobility.

At the expense of the GH joint's mobility comes a lack of stability. To maintain integrity, the joint relies upon a network of dynamic and static stabilizers. The dynamic stabilizers (named for their ability to move) are composed of the four rotator cuff muscles (supraspinatus, infraspinatus, teres minor, and subscapularis) (Fig. 8.2). In addition to enabling movements of the arm, the tendinous cuff formed by the common insertion of these muscles on the humeral head exerts a downward and inward force on the humerus, securing it snugly against the glenoid. The static stabilizers (referring to their inability to independently move) of the GH joint include the labrum, ligaments, joint capsule, and bony framework of the shoulder girdle.

BOX 8.1   The Golf Ball and the Seal's Nose

Although the title of this box sounds like the name of a children's book, it functions even better as a descriptor of the architecture of the shoulder joint. The articular surface of the humeral head is about three times as large as that of the glenoid fossa. As a result, a golf-ball-and-tee visual can help you compare the sizes of the humeral head (ball) and the glenoid fossa (tee). This analogy paints only a static picture, however. It is the ball-on-a-seal's-nose analogy that speaks to the glenohumeral joint's dynamics: A seal moves his nose to balance a ball, just like the muscles of the rotator cuff make microadjustments to keep the humeral head in constant contact with the glenoid fossa.

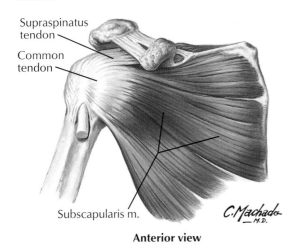

Supraspinatus tendon

Common tendon

Subscapularis m.

C. Machado —M.D.

Anterior view

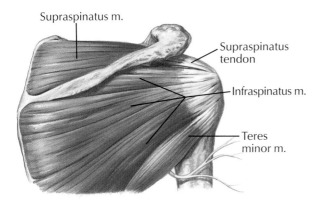

Supraspinatus m.

Supraspinatus tendon

Infraspinatus m.

Teres minor m.

Posterior view

Fig. 8.2 Rotator cuff: dynamic stabilizers of the glenohumeral joint.

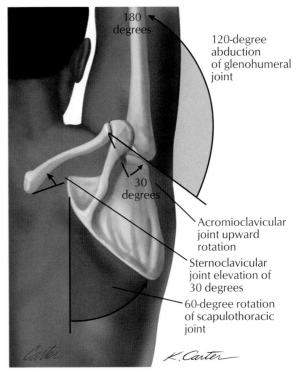

180 degrees

120-degree abduction of glenohumeral joint

30 degrees

Acromioclavicular joint upward rotation

Sternoclavicular joint elevation of 30 degrees

60-degree rotation of scapulothoracic joint

Carter

K. Carter

Fig. 8.3 Scapulohumeral rhythm.

MOVEMENT

With several joints and kinematic intricacies to study, it is easy to get lost in the details of the shoulder girdle. Instead, keep the big picture in mind and take note of how these joints often work in concert to enable movements of the arm and scapula. To execute arm flexion and abduction, for example, the joints move in a 2:1 ratio called scapulohumeral rhythm. For every 2 degrees of arm abduction, the scapula upwardly rotates 1 degree. Furthermore, because motion at the scapulothoracic joint results from coordination of the SC and AC joints, for every 2 degrees of scapular rotation, the SC elevates and the AC joint upwardly rotates by 1 degree each. Thus, the full 180-degree arc of arm movement from your torso to

your ear is actually the harmonious summation of 120 degrees of arm abduction and 60 degrees of scapular upward rotation (which, itself, is enabled by 30 degrees of SC joint elevation and 30 degrees of AC joint upward rotation) (Fig. 8.3).

MOVEMENT OF THE SCAPULOTHORACIC JOINT

Suspended mainly by muscles, and unencumbered by any true joint articulations, the scapula glides with ease across the posterior rib cage. Owing to the curved nature of the rib cage, the movements of the scapulothoracic (ST) joint occur as if around a sphere, and are categorized as (1) the more translational movements (including protraction [abduction], retraction [adduction], elevation, and depression), and (2) the rotatory movements, which help the scapula maintain contact with the thorax during arm movement and include rotation (upward and downward), winging (seen with winged scapula, see Clinical Focus 8.1), and tipping (anteriorly and posteriorly) (Fig. 8.4).

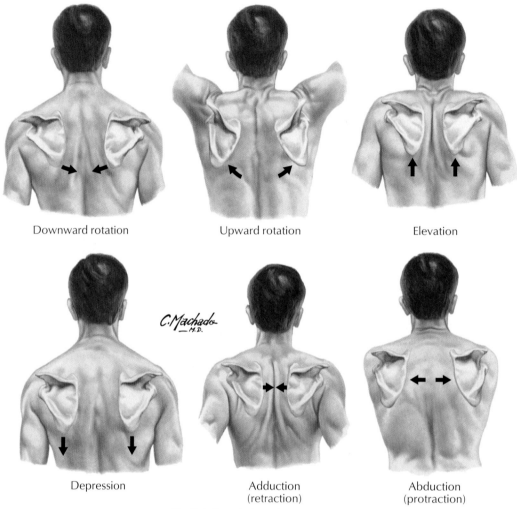

Fig. 8.4 Scapulothoracic movements.

Although they occur at the ST joint, these movements are not enabled by the ST joint alone. Common to both translational and rotatory movements is a reliance upon concurrent actions at the SC and AC joints; for example, as you abduct your arm and upwardly rotate your scapula, feel for yourself how your clavicle lifts (enabled by the SC and AC joints) in tandem. As such, the SC and AC joints work as a team to enable scapulothoracic movement, just as the coordination of all three joints (SC, AC, and ST) ensures proper functioning of the GH joint. The scapula, therefore, is one important piece of the much larger puzzle of the upper extremity, providing the foundation for how the shoulder, elbow, wrist, and hand move through space.

ELEVATION

Shrugging your shoulders is a classic example of scapular elevation. In this movement, the scapula slides superiorly along the posterior thorax, with the assistance of both the SC and AC joints. At the SC joint, the clavicle elevates; at the AC joint, the scapula subtly rotates downward enabling a fine-tuning motion that allows the scapula to remain nearly vertical as it rises (Practice What You Preach 8.1). Try **Moving AnatoME** with **Pilates Scapula Isolations** (Video 8.1), and notice how your scapular elevators "fire" to move your scapulae closer to your ears.

Approximate Range of Motion

45 degrees

Muscles and Innervation

See Fig. 8.5.

Muscle	Nerve
Trapezius (upper fibers)	Accessory nerve (cranial nerve XI) and C2-4
Levator scapulae	Dorsal scapular n. (C3-C5)
Rhomboid major and minor	Dorsal scapular n. (C4, C5)

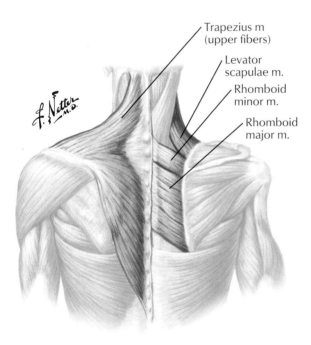

Trapezius m (upper fibers)
Levator scapulae m.
Rhomboid minor m.
Rhomboid major m.

Fig. 8.5 Muscles that elevate the scapula.

Moving AnatoME Exercise

Scapular Elevation: Pilates Scapula Isolations
See Fig. 8.6 and Video 8.1.

- Starting position: Lying supine on the floor. Your legs are hip distance apart, with knees flexed and feet flat on the floor. Arms extend by your sides with palms down. Abdominals are engaged, with navel drawing in toward the spine and lower ribs knitting together.
- Inhale to elevate the scapulae, gliding them along the mat.
- Exhale to depress the scapulae, gliding them along the mat.
- Repeat six to eight times.
- Ending position: Return the scapulae to a neutral position.

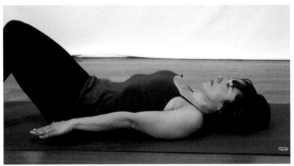

Fig. 8.6 Scapular elevation: **Pilates Scapula Isolations** (see Video 8.1).

DEPRESSION

If you shrug your shoulders up, you eventually need to lower them down. Scapular depression is responsible for the descent, moving the scapula inferiorly along the thorax. Its actions are the reverse of those of elevation. The SC joint depresses the clavicle, which permits the scapula to move inferiorly; the AC joint enables an upward rotation of the scapula to fine-tune the descent, allowing the scapula to remain nearly vertical as it is lowered (Practice What You Preach 8.2). Try **Moving AnatoME** with **Pilates Scapula Isolations** (see Video 8.1) to intentionally activate your scapular depressors and keep your shoulder girdle down, away from your ears.

Approximate Range of Motion

10 degrees

Muscles and Innervation

See Fig. 8.7.

Muscle	Nerve
Trapezius (lower fibers)	Accessory nerve (cranial nerve XI) and C2-4
Latissimus dorsi	Thoracodorsal n. (C6-C8)
Pectoralis minor	Medial pectoral n. (C8. T1)
Subclavius (via clavicle)	Nerve to subclavius (C5, C6)

PRACTICE WHAT YOU PREACH 8.2
The Antishrug

Without realizing it, you may be holding your shoulders in a perpetual shrug as you walk and text, hold a coffee cup, carry a heavy bag, or perform other activities. This regular scapular elevation can, over time, lead to neck tension, decreased range of motion, and muscular imbalances. To counteract a pervasive shrug and its untoward effects, practice the antishrug: Be aware of your scapulae throughout your day, and whenever they inch up toward your ears, activate your depressors to return your shoulder blades to a neutral position on your back.

Moving AnatoME Exercise
Scapular Depression: Pilates Scapula Isolations

See Fig. 8.8 and Video 8.1; see **Elevation** for exercise ◉ steps.

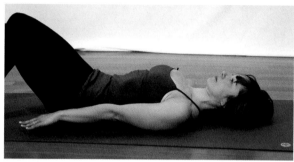

Fig. 8.8 Scapular depression: **Pilates Scapula Isolations** (see Video 8.1).

PROTRACTION

Perhaps you picked up this book from a table in front of you. If so, you protracted your scapula, a movement that permits forward reaching. Protraction moves the scapula away from the posterior midline of the body, a movement sometimes referred to as abduction. It is enabled by horizontal plane rotations at the SC and AC joints; the SC joint is responsible for the primary movement,

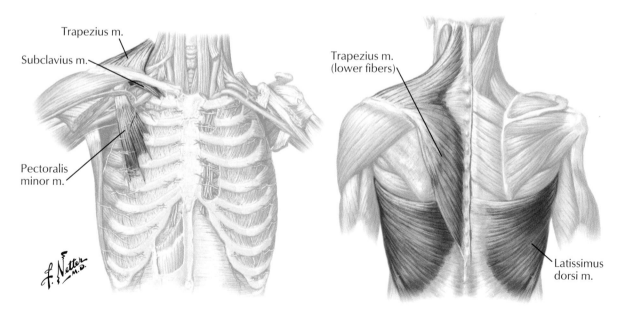

Fig. 8.7 Muscles that depress the scapula.

with the AC joint making microadjustments along the way. Protraction not only moves the scapula but can also help stabilize it. Stabilization is primarily imparted by the serratus anterior muscle, a scapular protractor that attaches to the medial border of the scapula; activating it not only protracts the scapula but also adheres it against the posterior thorax; this is an important feature of healthy upper extremity biomechanics (see winged scapula, Clinical Focus 8.1). Try **Moving AnatoME** with the **Yoga Cat-Cow Pose** (Video 8.2). In the cat position, feel the broadening of your back that occurs when you push your hands into the floor and activate your protractors.

Approximate Range of Motion

30 degrees

Muscles and Innervation

See Fig. 8.9.

Muscle	Nerve
Serratus anterior	Long thoracic n. (C5-C8)

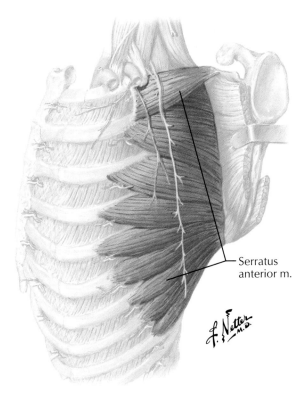

Fig. 8.9 Muscles that protract the scapula.

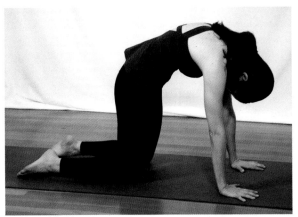

Fig. 8.10 Scapular protraction: **Yoga Cat-Cow Pose (Marjary-asana-Bitilasana)** (see Video 8.2).

Moving AnatoME Exercise

Scapular Protraction: Yoga Cat-Cow Pose (Marjaryasana-Bitilasana)
See Fig. 8.10, Video 8.2, and Clinical Focus 8.1.

- Starting position: In a quadruped position on your hands and knees, with wrists aligned under shoulders and knees under hips. The dorsa of your feet are flat on the floor. Your torso is parallel to the floor and your neck is neutral, with the gaze down and slightly in front of you.
- Enter into cat: On an exhale, flex your spine, reaching your head and sitting bones toward the floor. Simultaneously, press your hands and feet into the floor to encourage a rounding and lift of your thoracic spine toward the ceiling. As your hands press, feel your back broaden and scapulae protract. Make sure that there is no tension in your head and neck as they round toward the floor.
- Enter into cow: On the following inhale, extend your spine to lift your sitting bones and head. Isometrically pull your hands and knees toward one another to encourage the arch and opening of the front of the body. Feel your chest expand as your scapulae retract. Be mindful not to overextend your neck; it should follow the extension of the rest of the spine.
- Return to cat pose on the subsequent exhale, then cow on the inhale. Create a rhythmic flow as you move between the two poses.
- Cycle through five rounds of cat-cow.
- Ending position: Return to a neutral quadruped position.

CLINICAL FOCUS 8.1   **Winged Scapula**

A winged scapula is just that, a scapula with its medial border elevated off of the back, like a bird's wing. Normally, a scapula does not wing, because it is affixed to the posterior thoracic wall by muscles such as the serratus anterior. If muscle dysfunction occurs due to deconditioning or long thoracic nerve injury (ie, during a mastectomy), the scapula falls prey to unopposed muscular forces, resulting in its inferior angle tilting and its medial border flaring (eg, winging). Promote healthy shoulders with plank poses such as the **Pilates Push-Up** (see Video 9.1) to challenge your serratus anterior muscle. While in a plank position, resist the tendency to drop your rib cage toward the floor, resulting in a disengagement of your serratus anterior muscle and a winging of your scapula. Instead, stabilize and neutralize the scapula by gently pushing into the floor, inducing a subtle scapular protraction; this action engages, and thus strengthens, the serratus anterior muscle.

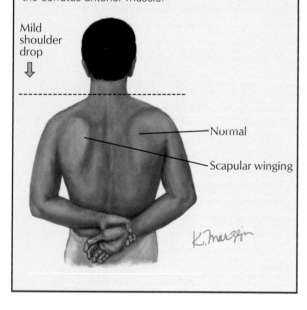

how your scapulae move toward the midline of your back. As you strengthen your scapular retractors, you are also stretching your anterior thoracic muscles.

Approximate Range of Motion

30 degrees

Muscles and Innervation

See Fig. 8.11.

Muscle	Nerve
Trapezius (middle fibers)	Accessory nerve (cranial nerve XI) and C2-4
Rhomboid major and minor	Dorsal scapular n. (C4, C5)

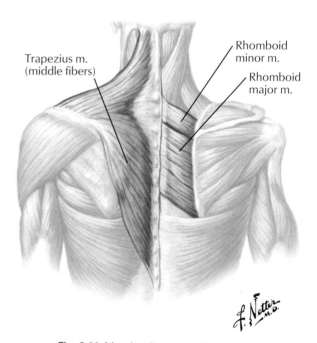

Fig. 8.11 Muscles that retract the scapula.

RETRACTION

After reaching for this book, you retract your scapulae to bring the book's pages within reading distance. Retraction draws the scapulae together, bringing them toward the midline of the body, a movement sometimes referred to as adduction. Like protraction, retraction employs SC and AC movement in the horizontal plane, but in the reverse direction. Try **Moving AnatoME** with **Yoga Cat-Cow Pose** (see Video 8.2). In the cat position, feel

Moving AnatoME Exercise

Scapular Retraction: Yoga Cat-Cow Pose (Marjaryasana-Bitilasana)

See Fig. 8.12 and Video 8.2; see **Protraction** for exercise steps.

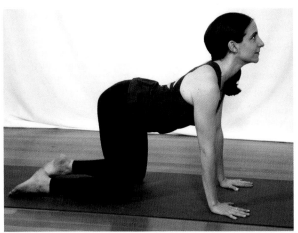

Fig. 8.12 Scapular retraction: **Yoga Cat-Cow Pose (Marjary-asana-Bitilasana)** (see Video 8.2)

UPWARD ROTATION

Your scapula rotates every time you raise your arm above your head. Why? When abducting or flexing the arm to bring it next to your ear, the humeral head can only go so far before bumping into the coracoacromial arch of the scapula. The scapula needs to upwardly rotate, therefore, to move the arch out of the way; when viewed posteriorly, this rotation moves the inferior angle of the scapula in a counterclockwise direction along the thorax, consequently providing more space for the humerus to move. With more space comes greater humeral abduction and, hence, a greater ability to lift your arm to your ear. As with all scapular movements, the SC and AC joints play a critical role; for 60 degrees of upward rotation of the scapula to occur, the SC joint allows 30 degrees of clavicular elevation and the AC joint allows for the remaining 30 degrees of upward scapular rotation. Try **Moving AnatoME** with a **Yoga Half Sun Salutation** (Video 8.3), and sense the movement of your scapulae on your back as they upwardly rotate to allow your arms to reach overhead.

Approximate Range of Motion

60 degrees

Muscles and Innervation

See Fig. 8.13.

Muscle	Nerve
Serratus anterior	Long thoracic n. (C5-C8)
Trapezius (upper, lower fibers)	Accessory nerve (cranial nerve XI) and C2-4

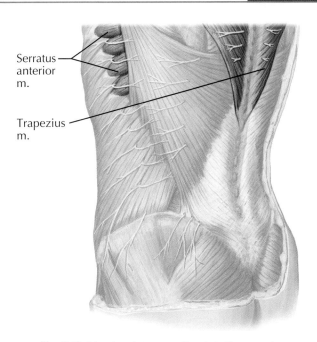

Fig. 8.13 Muscles that upwardly rotate the scapula.

Moving AnatoME Exercise
Scapular Upward Rotation: Yoga Half Sun Salutation

See Fig. 8.14 and Video 8.3.

- Starting position: Standing with your feet hip distance apart, in their natural parallel position. Weight is centered between both feet. Arms relax by your sides.
- Inhale, feel your scapulae stabilized on your back, externally rotate your shoulders and turn your palms anteriorly. Then abduct your arms overhead. Elevate your gaze as you raise your arms. If your flexibility allows, bring your palms together in a prayer position; otherwise, maintain parallel arms with palms facing each other. In either position, keep your shoulders depressed and away from the ears.
- Engage your core, and, on an exhale, adduct your arms as you simultaneously flex forward at the hips, lowering your torso toward the floor. Hands come to the floor, ankles, or shins. Head releases.
- Take a deep inhale and exhale, relaxing into the pose.
- On the next inhale, extend through the torso as you return to a standing position. Arms abduct as you rise, with your gaze elevating. As before, bring your palms to either a prayer pose or a parallel position.
- Exhale and adduct your arms to your sides, returning your head to neutral.

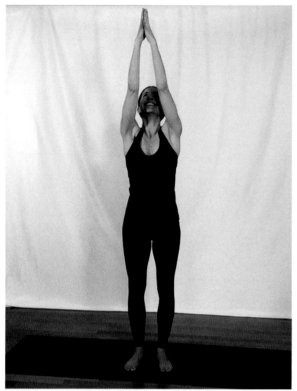

Fig. 8.14 Scapular upward rotation: **Yoga Half Sun Salutation** (see Video 8.3).

- Repeat for two more cycles.
- Ending position: Return to a neutral stance.

DOWNWARD ROTATION

If your arm is raised above your head, downward rotation of the scapula helps it return to your side. This motion is the converse of upward rotation (which helped raise your arm in the first place), with clavicular depression occurring at the SC joint while scapular downward rotation occurs at the AC joint. The movement is complete when the scapula is returned to its anatomical position. Try **Moving AnatoME** with a **Yoga Half Sun Salutation** (see Video 8.3), and sense the movement of your scapulae as they downwardly rotate to return your arms from overhead to your sides.

Approximate Range of Motion

From an upwardly rotated position (a range of motion of approximately 60 degrees), downward rotation returns the scapula to the anatomical position.

Muscles and Innervation

See Fig. 8.15.

Muscle	Nerve
Rhomboid major and minor	Dorsal scapular nerve (C4, C5)
Pectoralis minor	Medial pectoral nerve (C8.T1)
Latissimus dorsi	Thoracodorsal nerve (C6-C8)

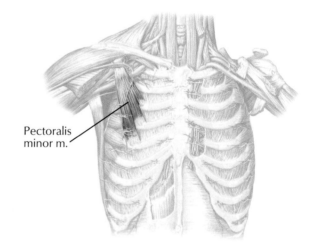

Pectoralis minor m.

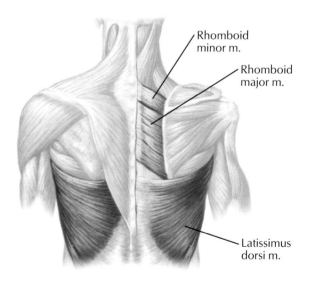

Rhomboid minor m.

Rhomboid major m.

Latissimus dorsi m.

Fig. 8.15 Muscles that downwardly rotate the scapula.

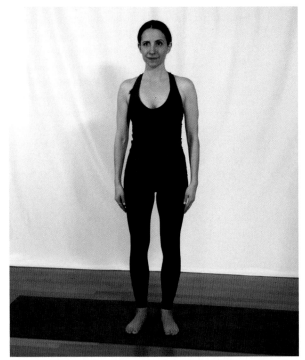

Fig. 8.16 Scapular downward rotation: **Yoga Half Sun Salutation** (see Video 8.3).

Moving AnatoME Exercise
Scapular Downward Rotation: Yoga Half Sun Salutation

▶ See Fig. 8.16 and Video 8.3; see **Upward Rotation** for exercise steps.

MOVEMENT OF THE GLENOHUMERAL (SHOULDER) JOINT

Whereas the ST joint facilitates movement of the scapula, the GH joint enables movement of the arm; it allows a wide range of movement, thanks to its distinctive golf ball-and-tee design. This architecture allows the humeral head to liberally glide and roll within the glenoid socket, enabling flexion, extension, abduction, adduction, and rotation of the arm (Fig. 8.17). Circumduction is also possible; it is the composite of the first four movements, experienced when you windmill your arms.

As with scapular movements, the arm movements enabled by the GH joint do not occur in isolation. Rather, the movements are coupled with one another *and* inextricably linked to the movements of the other shoulder

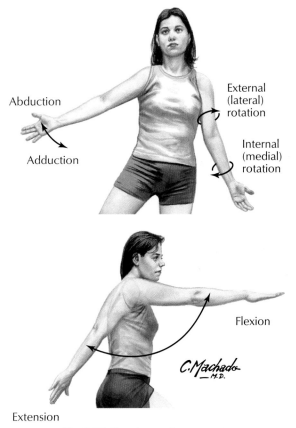

Fig. 8.17 Glenohumeral movements.

complex joints. For example, if you flex your right arm, a small amount of humeral internal rotation also occurs naturally. When learning movements of the GH joint, therefore, it is important to keep an eye on the bigger picture because there is no discrete point at which one motion ends and another begins.

FLEXION

You flex your arms every day when reaching for something high up on a shelf. During this motion, the head of the humerus spins posteriorly to move the arm anteriorly along the sagittal plane. Acting alone, the GH joint is responsible for about 120 degrees of flexion; upward rotation of the scapula is required to achieve the remaining 60 degrees. Try **Moving AnatoME** with the **Yoga Plank Pose** (Video 8.4). Form a stable foundation with your ▶ hands aligned directly under your shoulders so the arms are flexed at 90 degrees. To decrease weight bearing on

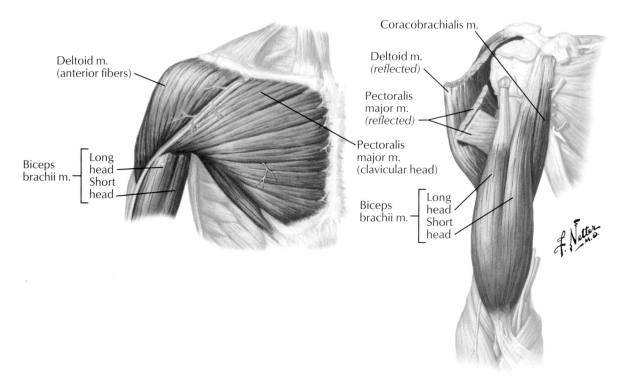

Fig. 8.18 Muscles that flex the shoulder.

the shoulder (and other upper extremity joints), modify the pose with the knees and/or forearms on the ground.

Approximate Range of Motion

120 degrees with only the GH joint involved; 180 degrees including scapular upward rotation.

Muscles and Innervation

See Fig. 8.18.

Muscle	Nerve
Deltoid (anterior fibers)	Axillary n. (C5, C6)
Pectoralis major (clavicular head)	Lateral and medial pectoral nn. (C5-T1)
Coracobrachialis	Musculocutaneous n. (C5-C7)
Biceps brachii	Musculocutaneous n. (C5, C6)

Moving AnatoME Exercise

Shoulder Flexion: Yoga Plank Pose (Phalakasana)

▶ See Fig. 8.19 and Video 8.4.

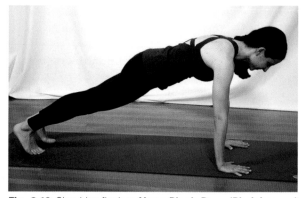

Fig. 8.19 Shoulder flexion: **Yoga Plank Pose (Phalakasana)** (see Video 8.4).

- Starting position: In a quadruped position on your hands and knees, with wrists aligned under shoulders and knees under hips. Your back is parallel to the floor, your core is engaged, and your neck is neutral, with your gaze down and slightly in front of you. Extend one leg behind you, dorsiflexing and reaching through the ankle, pressing your toes into the floor.

Bring the other leg into the same position to come into plank pose.

- Hold this plank position for five rounds of breath. Keep your core engaged to ensure that your lumbar spine does not hyperextend.
- Ending position: On an exhale, flex your elbows to lower your entire body—as a plank—slowly to the floor.

EXTENSION

After a long day, when you may have been hunched over as you worked, do you ever clasp your hands behind you to stretch your chest and shoulders? This arm position is extension. In a fashion similar to that of arm flexion, with extension, the humeral head spins anteriorly to move the arm posteriorly along the sagittal plane. With extension, however, the head of the humerus eventually meets resistance in the form of the anterior capsular ligaments, which prevent the arm from reaching more than 45 to 55 degrees behind the frontal plane; extension therefore

has a more limited range of movement. Of note, as the anterior capsular ligaments reach their maximum stretch, the scapula tips anteriorly very slightly, potentially lending a few extra degrees to the extension. Try **Moving AnatoME** with **Yoga Upward Plank Pose** (Video 8.5), and note how, with your arms in a fixed position, you isometrically engage your shoulder extensors. Your neck muscles should also be engaged but not tense.

Approximate Range of Motion
55 degrees

Muscles and Innervation
See Fig. 8.20.

Muscle	Nerve
Deltoid (posterior fibers)	Axillary nerve (C5, C6)
Latissimus dorsi	Thoracodorsal nerve (C6-C8)
Teres major	Lower subscapular nerve (C5, C6)

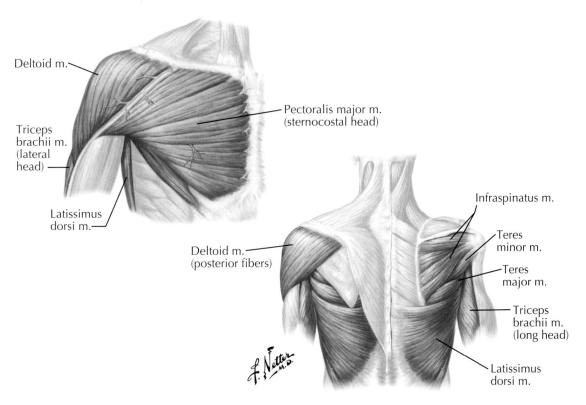

Fig. 8.20 Muscles that extend the shoulder.

Muscle	Nerve
Pectoralis major (sternocostal head)	Lateral and medial pectoral nerves (C5-T1)
Triceps brachii (long head)	Radial nerve (C6-C8)
Infraspinatus	Suprascapular nerve (C5, C6)
Teres minor	Axillary nerve (C5, C6)

Moving AnatoME Exercise

Shoulder Extension: Yoga Upward Plank Pose (Purvottanasana)

▶ See Fig. 8.21, Video 8.5, and Clinical Focus 8.2 and 8.3.

- Starting position: Sitting on the floor with legs extended in front of you, feet plantarflexed. If you need help maintaining an erect torso, place a cushion under your sitting bones. Arms are extended with palms on the floor a few inches behind your hips, fingertips pointing toward your feet.
- On an inhale, press your hands into and toes toward the floor to extend your hips and lift your pelvis. Bring your ankles, hips, shoulders, and ears into a diagonal line, from the floor to the ceiling; nod your chin to lengthen and protect the neck. (If you are unable to enter this position, flex your knees and place your feet flat on the floor to come into a reverse quadruped position for the duration of the exercise.)
- Stabilize your shoulders and scapulae to support the extension of your thoracic spine. Extend the hips to lift your pelvis, without gripping your buttocks.

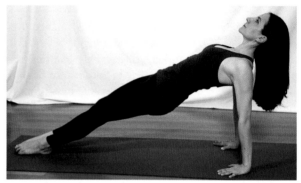

Fig. 8.21 Shoulder extension: **Yoga Upward Plank Pose (Purvottanasana)** (see Video 8.5).

CLINICAL FOCUS 8.2   Shoulder Instability

Shoulder instability encompasses a group of conditions (laxity, subluxation, and dislocation) related to pathologic hypermobility of the glenohumeral joint. In each of these hypermobile states, the humeral head loses contact with the glenoid fossa; it is the degree of contact loss and severity of symptoms that distinguishes each entity, with dislocation being the most severe. Individuals with shoulder instability should be cautious when exercising in relatively unstable shoulder positions, such as extension. To be safe, the shoulder should be strengthened in more stable positions, such as adduction and flexion, as seen with the **Yoga Plank Pose** (see Video 8.4); modifying the pose with knees placed on the ground further decreases stress on the joint.

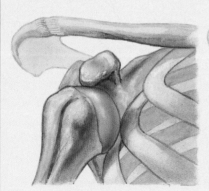
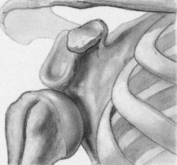
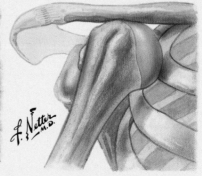

Subcoracoid dislocation (most common)   Subglenoid dislocation   Subclavicular dislocation (uncommon)

CLINICAL FOCUS 8.3 Shoulder Separation

Although the term *shoulder separation* sounds similar to *shoulder instability*, the former is a distinct pathology occurring at a different joint. Whereas instability affects the glenohumeral joint, shoulder separation involves a disruption of the stabilizing ligaments of the acromioclavicular joint. With injured ligaments, this superficial joint further loses integrity, and its articulating bones may become displaced. A separation often results from trauma, such as a superior blow to the shoulder during a football tackle or a lateral blow to the shoulder during a hockey check into a wall. For individuals with a mild shoulder separation, early mobility is imperative to prevent stiffening of the shoulder and possible progression to adhesive capsulitis (see Clinical Focus 8.6). Gentle stretches used for adhesive capsulitis, such as arm circles, can also be used with mild shoulder separations.

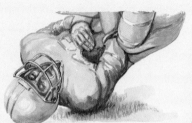
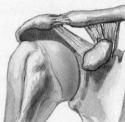
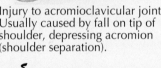
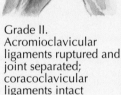
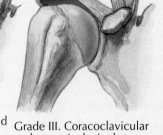
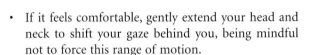

Injury to acromioclavicular joint. Usually caused by fall on tip of shoulder, depressing acromion (shoulder separation).

Grade I. Acromioclavicular ligaments stretched but not torn; coracoclavicular ligaments intact

Grade II. Acromioclavicular ligaments ruptured and joint separated; coracoclavicular ligaments intact

Grade III. Coracoclavicular and acromioclavicular ligaments ruptured, with wide separation of joint

- If it feels comfortable, gently extend your head and neck to shift your gaze behind you, being mindful not to force this range of motion.
- Breathe for five rounds.
- Ending position: Return your head to neutral, flex your hips, and slowly lower your buttocks to a seated position.

ABDUCTION

Perform the first half of a jumping jack—with arms raised high, palms touching above the head—for a very simple example of arm abduction. The movement of abduction, however, is anything but:

- **From 0 to 90 degrees**: Abduction at the GH joint occurs as the head of the humerus rolls superiorly and slides inferiorly on the glenoid fossa, to move the arm along the frontal plane. This combined roll-and-slide movement prevents the head from jamming into the acromion, thereby preventing impingement of the supraspinatus tendon (see Clinical Focus 8.4, Impingement Syndrome). The GH joint is helped at approximately 30 degrees, when scapular upward rotation and clavicular elevation begin.
- **From 90 to 150 degrees**: At about 90 degrees, the limit of GH abduction is reached, and clavicular elevation ends. For abduction to proceed, muscles such as the serratus anterior must upwardly rotate the scapula a total of 60 degrees (30 degrees by the SC joint and 30 degrees by the AC joint).
- **From 150 to 180 degrees**: Abduction beyond 150 degrees requires some motion at the vertebral joints of the cervical spine and upper thorax; bilateral abduction requires that the thoracic and lumbar spines extend.

Of note, the GH joint is capable of horizontal abduction, as well, a movement named for what it does: abduction of the humerus with the arm moving medially to laterally along a transverse plane (ie, with the shoulder flexed to 90 degrees). Try **Moving AnatoME** with the **Pilates Side Arm Series (Abduction)** (Video 8.6). For greater emphasis and strengthening, use a resistance band or create your own resistance and move your arms as if they were in water.

Approximate Range of Motion

120 degrees with only the GH joint involved; 180 degrees including scapular upward rotation.

Muscles and Innervation

See Fig. 8.22.

Muscle	Nerve
Deltoid (anterior and middle fibers; posterior fibers involved in horizontal abduction)	Axillary n. (C5, C6)
Supraspinatus	Suprascapular n. (C5, C6)

Moving AnatoME Exercise

Shoulder Abduction: Pilates Side Arm Series (Abduction)

See Fig. 8.23, Video 8.6, and Clinical Focus 8.4 and 8.5.
- Starting position: Kneeling on the floor atop of a resistance band so that there are equal band lengths on either side of you. Knees are hip width apart, hips stack over knees, core is engaged, and shoulders stack over hips.
- With each hand, grab onto an end of the resistance band, keeping your palms facing forward.
- Inhale and engage your core.
- Exhale, stabilize your torso, and abduct both arms to 180 degrees, pulling against the resistance of the band.

Keep the scapulae stabilized throughout the range of motion, gently depressing them away from your ears as they upwardly rotate to allow the full range of motion.
- At 180 degrees, your palms should face one another.
- Inhale and slowly adduct the arms, downwardly rotating the scapulae. Control the motion by resisting the pull of gravity as you lower your hands back to your sides.
- Repeat six to eight times.
- Ending position: Release the band and relax the arms by your sides.

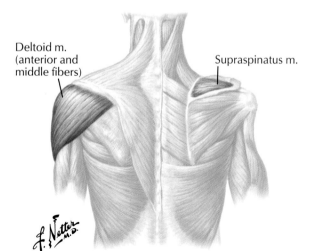

Deltoid m. (anterior and middle fibers)

Supraspinatus m.

Fig. 8.22 Muscles that abduct the shoulder.

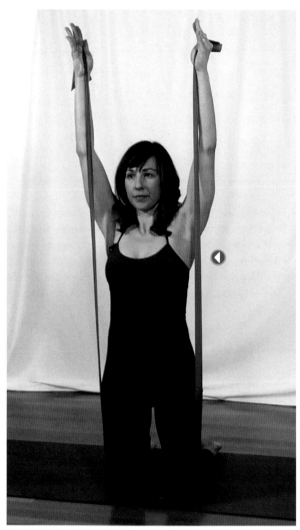

Fig. 8.23 Shoulder abduction: **Pilates Side Arm Series (Abduction)** (see Video 8.6).

CLINICAL FOCUS 8.4 Impingement Syndrome

The term *impingement syndrome* refers to a range of damage and dysfunction related to soft tissue structures of the subacromial space, the narrow, bony area between the head of the humerus and the underside of the acromion. The supraspinatus tendon, as well as the subacromial bursa, are in this tight space. Add in common problems that further decrease the size of the interval, such as weak rotator cuff muscles, anatomical anomalies, degeneration of structures, or repetitive overhead motions, and rotator cuff havoc ensues. Caught between a rock and a hard place, the tendons and bursa are prone to repetitive microtrauma, ultimately leading to bursitis, tendinitis, and rotator cuff tears. The impact of this syndrome is far-reaching, affecting a wide range of individuals from overusers (eg, athletes) to underusers (eg, the elderly). Impingement is exacerbated by movements that further decrease the subacromial space (eg, abduction, flexion). While one is recovering from this condition, therefore, the range of motion in exercises that incorporate these

movements should be modified. For example, in the **Yoga Tree Pose** (see Video 13.1), keep your hands in prayer position next to the sternum, in lieu of elevating them overhead to minimize the flexion.

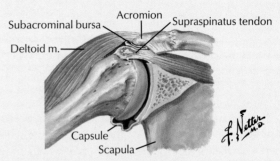

Abduction of arm causes repeated impingement of greater tubercle of humerus on acromion, leading to degeneration and inflammation of supraspinatus tendon, secondary inflammation of bursa, and pain on abduction of arm.

CLINICAL FOCUS 8.5 Rotator Cuff Injury

The inherent hypermobility of the shoulder takes its toll on the joint's dynamic stabilizers, the rotator cuff muscles. In fact, rotator cuff injuries are a frequent cause of shoulder problems, manifesting as a tearing or inflammation of one or more of the rotator cuff tendons. Tendon tears can be partial or complete, and the supraspinatus is the most frequently injured. Due to its location beneath the bony acromion, just

inferior to the subacromial bursa, its tendon is particularly susceptible to wear and tear. Common causes of tears include impingement syndrome (see Clinical Focus 8.4), trauma, and deconditioning. Prevent this common injury by keeping the rotator cuff muscles healthy with regular, light resistance (eg, from a flex band), as experienced with the **Pilates Side Arm Series** (see Videos 8.6 and 8.7).

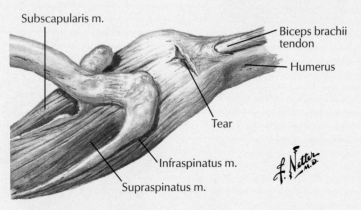

Acute rupture (superior view). Often associated with splitting tear parallel to tendon fibers.

ADDUCTION

To complete the jumping jack from the prior example: slap your hands on your thighs by adducting your arms. Adduction is biomechanically easier than abduction; for the initial 180 to 120 degrees, the scapula downwardly rotates to make space for the humeral head. The humeral head, in its descent, rolls inferiorly and slides superiorly on the glenoid fossa to move the arm along the frontal plane.

Horizontal adduction is a subset of adduction, occurring when the arm moves laterally to medially across the body following a transverse plane (ie, with the shoulder flexed to 90 degrees).

Try **Moving AnatoME** with **Pilates Side Arm Series (Adduction)** (see Video 8.6). Lower your arms with resistance against gravity to enhance the strengthening of your adductor muscles.

Approximate Range of Motion

From a fully abducted position (a range of motion of approximately 180 degrees), adduction returns the arm to the anatomical position.

Muscles and Innervation

See Fig. 8.24.

Muscle	Nerve
Triceps brachii (long head)	Radial n. (C6-C8)
Latissimus dorsi	Thoracodorsal n. (C6-C8)
Teres major	Lower subscapular n. (C5, C6)
Pectoralis major (sternocostal head; clavicular head involved in horizontal adduction)	Lateral and medial pectoral nn. (C5-T1)
Infraspinatus	Suprascapular n. (C5, C6)
Teres minor	Axillary n.(C5, C6)
Deltoid (posterior fibers)	Axillary n.(C5, C6)

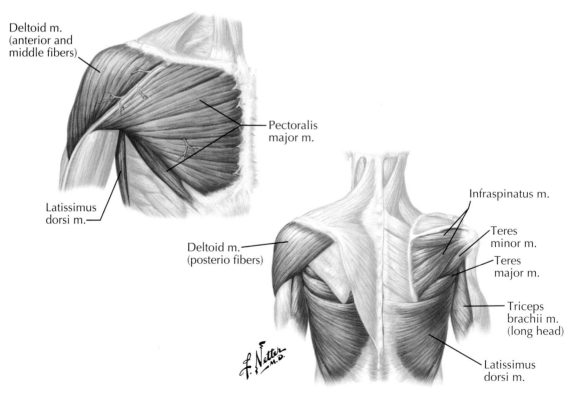

Fig. 8.24 Muscles that adduct the shoulder.

Moving AnatoME Exercise
Shoulder Adduction: Pilates Side Arm
Series (Adduction)

See Fig. 8.25 and Video 8.6. See **Abduction** for exercise steps.

a longitudinal axis of rotation, with the anterior surface of the shaft revolving laterally, away from the midline. Try **Moving AnatoME** with the **Pilates Side Arm Series (External Rotation)** (Video 8.7) and be mindful not to let the elbow drift away from your rib cage (a common mistake) in order to isolate pure external rotation.

Approximate Range of Motion

70 degrees; in a position of 90 degrees of abduction, external rotation may increase to 90 degrees.

Muscles and Innervation

See Fig. 8.26.

Muscle	Nerve
Infraspinatus	Suprascapular n. (C5, C6)
Teres minor	Axillary n. (C5, C6)
Deltoid (posterior fibers)	Axillary n. (C5, C6)

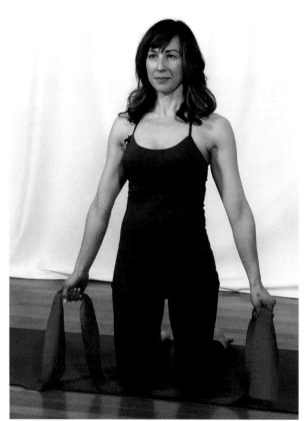

Fig. 8.25 Shoulder adduction: **Pilates Side Arm Series (Adduction)** (see Video 8.6).

EXTERNAL ROTATION

Think about how you throw a baseball and use the "wind-up" motion, which includes a large external rotation, that occurs just before the pitch. In order to externally rotate, the head of the humerus rolls posteriorly and slides anteriorly on the glenoid fossa, which acts as a platform; the roll-plus-slide movement allows the much larger humeral head to move over a smaller glenoid fossa. The humeral shaft simultaneously revolves around

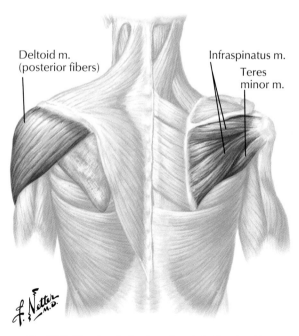

Deltoid m.
(posterior fibers)

Infraspinatus m.
Teres
minor m.

Fig. 8.26 Muscles that externally rotate the shoulder.

Moving AnatoME Exercise
Shoulder External Rotation: Pilates Side Arm Series (External Rotation)

See Fig. 8.27, Video 8.7, and Clinical Focus 8.6.

- Starting position: Sitting in a cross-legged position on the floor. Sit in the middle of the band so that there are equal band lengths on either side of you (sit on a cushion or a rolled-up edge of your mat if you need help sitting erect atop of your sitting bones).

- With your right hand, grab the opposite band; flex and supinate your right elbow and adduct your right shoulder to bring the forearm parallel to the ground, making a 90-degree angle.
- Inhale and engage your core.
- Exhale, stabilize your torso, and externally rotate your right shoulder, pulling against the resistance of the band. Keep your shoulder adducted and your elbow alongside your torso. Only rotate as far as you can maintain a neutral spine and pelvis.

CLINICAL FOCUS 8.6   Adhesive Capsulitis

The nickname of this condition, frozen shoulder, says it all. An immobilizing condition, adhesive capsulitis results from an inflammation, thickening, and contraction of the glenohumeral joint capsule. The condition is idiopathic and generally afflicts middle-aged women. It usually begins as a progressive loss of both active and passive shoulder mobility, and it eventually results in incapacitating pain. Much about its pathogenesis is still unknown, but there is a capsular fibrosis and shortening associated with movement loss, which predominantly limits external rotation, flexion, abduction, and internal rotation. Early range-of-motion therapy is therefore important to reintroduce mobility. Doing simple, gentle arm circles within a pain-free range of motion, and performed on the floor if necessary, is a good place to start.

Markedly limited active and passive motion, right shoulder. All planes of shoulder motion restricted and painful at extremes.

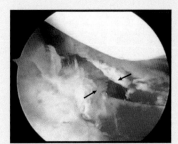

Intraarticular findings of synovitis and loss of capsular volume, as well as the arthroscopic releases (arrows) performed with arthroscopic surgery.

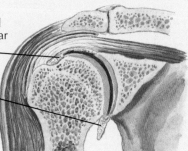

Adhesions of peripheral capsule to distal articular cartilage

Adhesions obliterating axillary fold of capsule

Coronal section of shoulder shows adhesions between capsule and periphery of humeral head.

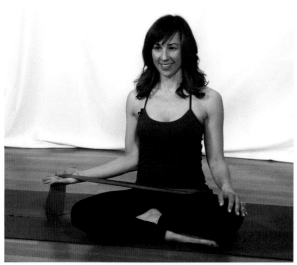

Fig. 8.27 Shoulder external rotation: **Pilates Side Arm Series (External Rotation)** (see Video 8.7).

- Inhale and internally rotate the right shoulder, keeping the forearm parallel to the ground as you bring the forearm closer to the torso, slowly controlling the release of tension in the band.
- Repeat six to eight times, and then repeat the exercise on the other arm.
- Ending position: Release the band and relax the arms by your sides.

INTERNAL ROTATION

When swimming the breaststroke, internal rotation of your shoulders plays a major part in the pull-through phase of the stroke, propelling you quickly through the water. Internal rotation is the movement opposite to external rotation. With internal rotation, the head of the humerus rolls anteriorly and slides posteriorly on the glenoid fossa, preventing unsafe anterior displacement of the humeral head. As with external rotation, the humeral shaft subsequently revolves around a longitudinal axis of rotation in the opposite direction, with the anterior surface of the shaft revolving medially, toward the midline. Try **Moving AnatoME** with the **Pilates Side Arm Series (Internal Rotation)** (see Video 8.7), making sure to keep your elbow in contact with your torso to properly isolate the internal rotator muscles.

Range of Motion

85 degrees

Muscles and Innervation

See Fig. 8.28.

Muscle	Nerve
Deltoid (anterior fibers)	Axillary n. (C5, C6)
Subscapularis	Upper and lower subscapular nn. (C5, C6)
Latissimus dorsi	Thoracodorsal n. (C6-C8)
Teres major	Lower subscapular n. (C5, C6)
Pectoralis major	Lateral and medial pectoral nn. (C5-T1)

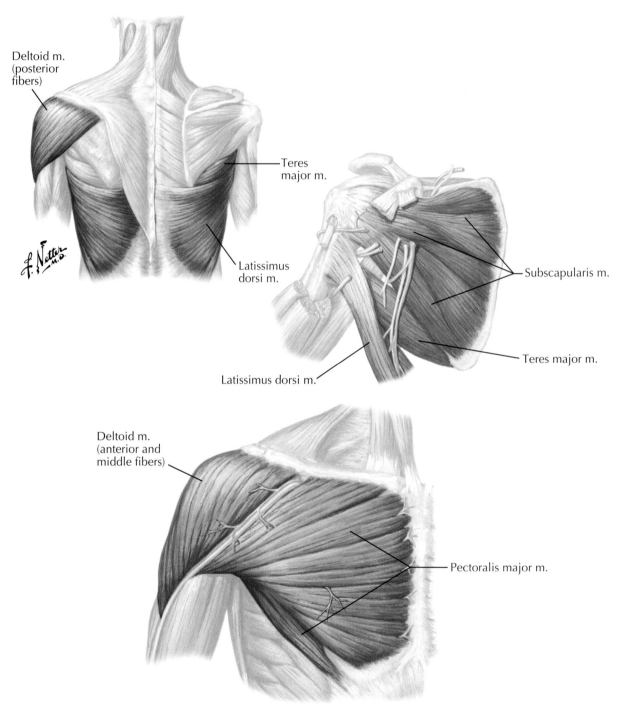

Fig. 8.28 Muscles that internally rotate the scapula.

Moving AnatoME Exercise

Shoulder Internal Rotation: Pilates Side Arm Series (Internal Rotation)

See Fig. 8.29 and Video 8.7. See **External Rotation** for exercise steps.

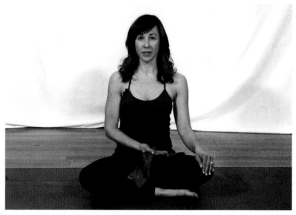

Fig. 8.29 Shoulder internal rotation: **Pilates Side Arm Series (Internal Rotation)** (see Video 8.7).

9

Elbow

OVERVIEW

- The elbow is a modified hinge joint that connects the arm and forearm. It is closely associated with the joints of the forearm.
- Its articulations occur between the humerus and ulna (the humeroulnar joint), humerus and radius (the humeroradial joint), and radius and ulna (the proximal radioulnar joint). The latter joint is one of the three radioulnar joints of the forearm (proximal, middle, and distal).
- Movements include flexion and extension (at the humeroulnar and humeroradial joints), as well as pronation and supination (at the radioulnar joints).
- Example exercises:
  - Flexion (**Pilates Push-Up,** Video 9.1)
  - Extension (**Pilates Push-Up,** Video 9.1)
  - Supination (**Yoga Cow Face Pose,** Video 9.2)
  - Pronation (**Yoga Cow Face Pose,** Video 9.2)

STRUCTURE AND FUNCTION

When you bang an elbow, you may say you've hit your funny bone (and will feel an *un*funny tingling sensation radiating into your forearm and hand). However, the funny "bone" reference is erroneous; the sensation you experience from banging your elbow is not from compression of a bone but, rather, of the ulnar nerve, which wraps superficially around the ulna.

The ulna is one of the bones that forms the elbow joint. Although it is classified as a single synovial hinge joint, the elbow is actually the composite of three separate articulations between (Fig. 9.1A)

1. The trochlear notch of the ulna and the trochlea of the humerus (the humeroulnar joint);

2. the head of the radius and the capitulum of the humerus (the humeroradial joint); and,
3. the head of the radius and the radial notch of the ulna (proximal radioulnar joint).

One synovial cavity houses the articular surfaces, which are encased by hyaline cartilage. A large capsule lined with a synovial membrane, and fortified by medial and lateral collateral ligaments, encloses and stabilizes the joint (see Fig. 9.1B).

The articulations that connect the humerus to the ulna and radius are the primary movers of the joint, permitting extension and flexion of the forearm. Even though the elbow is usually classified as a typical hinge joint, these articulations functionally resemble ball-and-socket structures. The humeral trochlea acts as the ball and the ulnar trochlear notch as the socket; in conjunction, the capitulum of the humerus and the fovea of the radius act as a miniature ball-and-socket joint.

The proximal radioulnar joint works with its middle and distal radioulnar counterparts to pronate and supinate the forearm. Additionally, the middle radioulnar joint transmits force via its syndesmotic connection, which includes an interosseous membrane joining the radius and ulna. The distal radioulnar joint, a synovial joint located closer to the wrist (but part of the forearm), also shares forces incurred by the forearm.

This system of joints works together as the elbow-forearm complex, to move the forearm through uniplanar motion (ie, flexion and extension), as well as rotation (ie, pronation and supination) (see Fig. 9.2). Envision a baseball pitcher winding up and then throwing the ball to contextualize how much hand movement, and range of placement, this system of joints is able to provide. In your own life, the four movements allow you to hold a tray of soup 2 feet in front of you or pick up your keys from the floor 2 feet behind you (Clinical Focus 9.1).

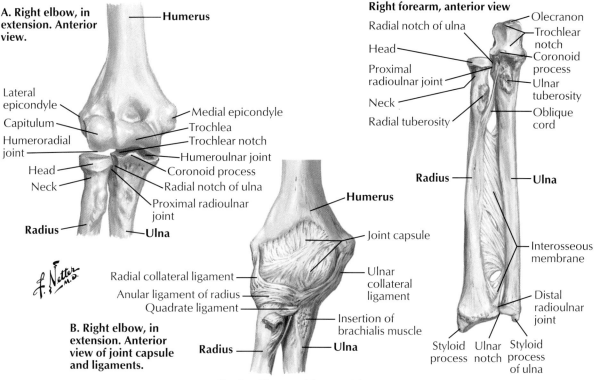

A. Right elbow, in extension. Anterior view.

Humerus

Lateral epicondyle
Capitulum
Humeroradial joint
Head
Neck
Radius
Ulna
Medial epicondyle
Trochlea
Trochlear notch
Humeroulnar joint
Coronoid process
Radial notch of ulna
Proximal radioulnar joint

B. Right elbow, in extension. Anterior view of joint capsule and ligaments.

Radial collateral ligament
Anular ligament of radius
Quadrate ligament
Radius

Humerus
Joint capsule
Ulnar collateral ligament
Insertion of brachialis muscle
Ulna

Right forearm, anterior view

Radial notch of ulna
Head
Proximal radioulnar joint
Neck
Radial tuberosity
Radius
Ulna

Olecranon
Trochlear notch
Coronoid process
Ulnar tuberosity
Oblique cord
Interosseous membrane
Distal radioulnar joint

Styloid process Ulnar notch Styloid process of ulna

Fig. 9.1 Elbow and forearm joints.

MOVEMENT

Compared with the multitude of movements performed by the arm, forearm biomechanics may seem simple; they consist of flexion, extension, supination, and pronation (Fig. 9.2). Yet they are integral to many everyday functions, such as lifting a glass so you can drink water, pushing a door open, brushing your hair, and reaching into a refrigerator. They permit our hands to be placed in a variety of positions. They can also be performed with either a free forearm (as seen with a dumbbell curl) or a fixed forearm (as seen with a push-up). Although both types of movements are important (open-chain and closed-chain, respectively), this chapter focuses on the open-chain movements, which are more regularly performed by the upper extremity.

FLEXION

Did you brush your teeth this morning? If so, thank flexion of the forearm—a simple but profoundly important elbow movement—for your pearly whites. When the arm flexors contract, they pull the forearm closer to the arm, rolling and sliding the ulnar trochlear notch around the trochlea of the humerus; the radial fovea and capitulum of the humerus mimic the same action, respectively. Try **Moving AnatoME** with **Pilates Push-Up** (Video 9.1). As you lower your torso to the floor, control the flexion of your forearms for a smooth descent, instead of succumbing to gravity (Practice What You Preach 9.1).

Approximate Range of Motion

145 degrees; daily activities typically use a more limited range of 30 to 130 degrees

Muscles and Innervation

See Fig. 9.3.

Muscle	Nerve
Brachialis	Musculocutaneous n. (C5, C6)
Biceps brachii	Musculocutaneous n. (C5, C6)
Brachioradialis	Radial n. (C5, C6)
Pronator teres	Median n. (C6, C7)

CLINICAL FOCUS 9.1
Lateral and Medial Epicondylitis

Epicondylitis is a common overuse injury typically felt near the elbow but affecting forearm muscles that move the wrist. Repetitive use of these muscles can damage the tendons near their insertion points, resulting in signs and symptoms associated degeneration (eg, tenderness, pain). Lateral epicondylitis (the most prevalent form) involves tendons of the wrist extensor muscles near their origins on the lateral humeral epicondyle. It is also known as *tennis elbow* because repetitive use of these muscles by tennis players gives them a propensity to develop the injury. In comparison, medial epicondylitis afflicts the common flexor tendon near the medial humeral epicondyle. It is known as *golfer's elbow* because golfers rely on and may overuse the wrist flexor muscles. Flexible forearm muscles are key to preventing these overuse injuries, which commonly occur in middle-aged recreational athletes and others who engage in activities utilizing repetitive forearm motion (eg, carpentry). Keep the forearms supple with a daily "dose" of wrist circles (performed in both directions); progress to the **Yoga Hand-to-Foot Pose** (see Video 10.1) and **Yoga Prayer Position** (see Video 11.3) to stretch the extensors and flexors, respectively.

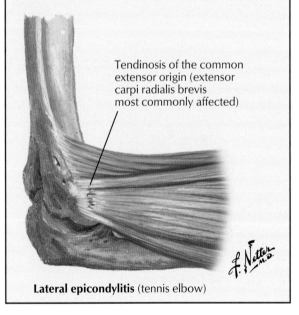

Tendinosis of the common extensor origin (extensor carpi radialis brevis most commonly affected)

Lateral epicondylitis (tennis elbow)

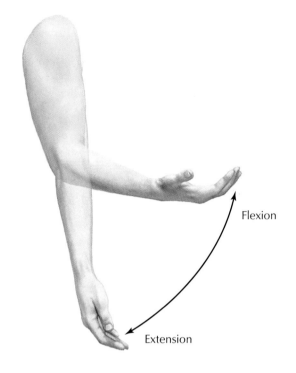

Flexion

Extension

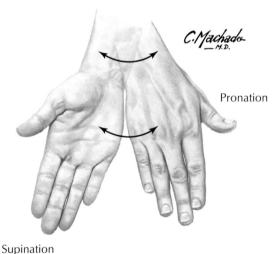

Pronation

Supination

Fig. 9.2 Elbow movements.

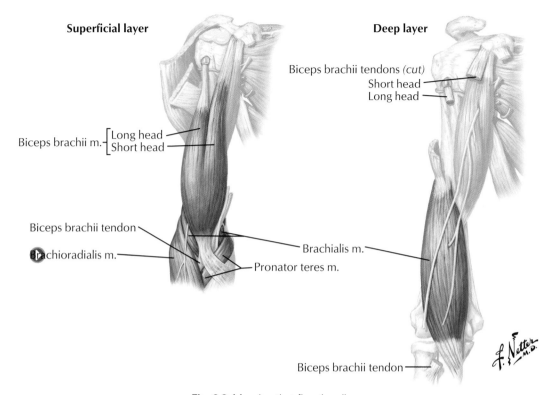

Superficial layer

Biceps brachii m. ⎡Long head
              ⎣Short head

Biceps brachii tendon

Brachioradialis m.

Brachialis m.

Pronator teres m.

Deep layer

Biceps brachii tendons *(cut)*
Short head
Long head

Biceps brachii tendon

Fig. 9.3 Muscles that flex the elbow.

PRACTICE WHAT YOU PREACH 9.1
When Studying Is a Hazard to Your Health

While your brain flourishes in school, your elbows and forearms take a beating. You lean on flexed elbows to prop your head up in class, and your forearm muscles work overtime to furiously text, type, and scribble notes. When repeated daily, these mild assaults can wreak chronic havoc, leaving you with forms of lateral and medial epicondylitis (see Clinical Focus 9.1). To avoid these studying hazards, bring awareness to your posture. Depend less on your elbows and more on sleep and a strong core to keep you upright in class. And, after class is done, relieve your forearm muscles with a short self-massage, as well as wrist circles (in both directions).

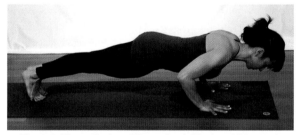

Fig. 9.4 Elbow flexion: **Pilates Push-Up** (see Video 9.1).

BOX 9.1   Two Heads, Two Roles

Thanks in part to the cartoon character Popeye, the biceps brachii muscle is thought of as a forearm flexor. But it is actually a much more powerful forearm supinator. This role is so important that the biceps brachii muscle performs its flexing functions best when the forearm is supinated; this is why a chin-up (with forearms supinated) is much easier to do than a pull-up (with forearms pronated).

Moving AnatoME Exercise
Elbow Flexion: Pilates Push-Up
See Fig. 9.4, Video 9.1, and Box 9.1.

- Starting position: In a plank position (see Video 8.4) with hands underneath the shoulders and elbows extended. Press into the floor to mildly protract and stabilize the scapulae on the back. Engage your core and keep your spine as neutral as possible with slight lumbar flexion. Extend your hips and knees and dorsiflex your ankles, pressing the base of each toe into the floor. Reach through your heels, forming one long line from your heels through your knees, hips, shoulders, and ears. (Lower your knees to the floor for a modification.)

- Inhale, flex the elbows, while you extend and abduct the shoulders so the elbows reach out at a 45-degree angle to your body. Lower down on three counts, stabilizing the scapulae on the back and maintaining a neutral spine. Lower down only as far as you can maintain a neutral spine.
- Exhale, engage your core, and extend your elbows to return to the starting position.
- Repeat six to eight times.
- Ending position: On the final exhale, flex your elbows to lower your entire body—as a plank—slowly to the floor.

EXTENSION

When you push "up" during a push-up, you extend your forearms. This movement, which increases the distance between the anterior arm and the forearm, happens in the reverse direction of flexion. As the angle between the arm and forearm increases, the ulnar trochlea moves within the humeral trochlear notch and the fovea of the radius rolls and slides within the humeral capitulum. Note that in anatomical position, the elbows rest in an extended position; extension past this neutral posture is limited by the bony articulation between the olecranon and olecranon fossa, as well as increased tension in the surrounding capsule, ligaments, and flexor muscles. (see Fig. 9.1). Try **Moving AnatoME** with a **Pilates Push-Up** (see Video 9.1). When you push up, feel your triceps work against gravity to extend your forearms. On the descent, likewise notice how your triceps work eccentrically to control your motion.

Approximate Range of Motion

5 degrees of hyperextension

Muscles and Innervation

See Fig. 9.5.

Muscle	Nerve
Triceps brachii	Radial n. (C6-C8)
Anconeus	Radial n. (C7-T1)

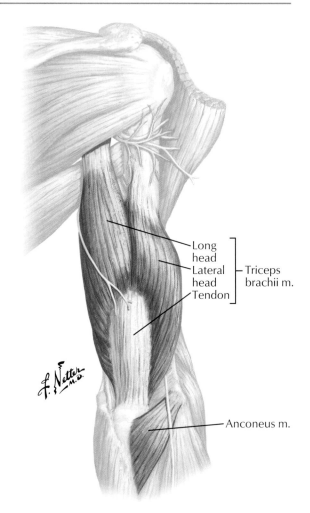

Fig. 9.5 Muscles that extend the elbow. (Muscles not shown: medial head of triceps brachii, lies deep.)

Moving AnatoME Exercise

Elbow Extension: Pilates Push-Up

See Fig. 9.6 and Video 9.1; see **Flexion** for exercise steps.

SUPINATION

To carry a tray with *soup*, you need to *sup*inate. Supination is the rotation of the anterior surface of the forearm laterally; it occurs between the radioulnar joints, with the radius rotating around a stationary ulna. At the proximal radioulnar joint, the radial head spins within the radial notch of the ulna; at the distal radioulnar joint, the ulnar notch of the radius rolls and slides on the head

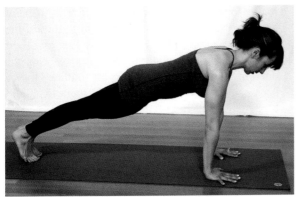

Fig. 9.6 Elbow extension: **Pilates Push-Up** (see Video 9.1).

of the ulna. Additionally, the interosseous membrane (acting as the middle joint) connects the two to create a uniform movement, as well as transmit force. The direction of the spin, roll, and slide is the same as the direction of the moving thumb. Notice that it is impossible to supinate beyond a certain extent; this limitation is due to many factors including the finite stretch of the palmar capsule ligament, the presence of the interosseous membrane, and the connective tissue structures of the ulnocarpal complex (see Figs. 9.1 and 10.1). Try **Moving AnatoME** with **Yoga Cow Face Pose** (Video 9.2). Note that your top forearm is supinated. If you are unable to hold hands, hold a towel, or your shirt, to maintain the connection between and proper positioning of your forearms.

Approximate Range of Motion
85 degrees (individuals with a decreased range may compensate by externally rotating at the shoulder)

Muscles and Innervation
See Figs. 9.7 and 9.3 (for biceps brachii).

Muscle	Nerve
Biceps brachii	Musculocutaneous n. (C5, C6)
Supinator	Deep branch of radial n. (C5, C6)
Extensor pollicis longus	Posterior interosseous n. (C7, C8)
Extensor indicis	Posterior interosseous n. (C7, C8)

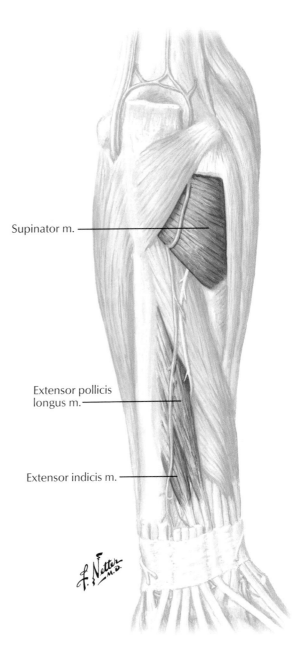

Fig. 9.7 Muscles that supinate the forearm.

Moving AnatoME Exercises
Elbow Supination: Yoga Cow Face Pose (Gomukhasana)
See Fig. 9.8 and Video 9.2.
- Starting position: Sitting on the floor with legs extended in front of you, feet dorsiflexed. If you need help

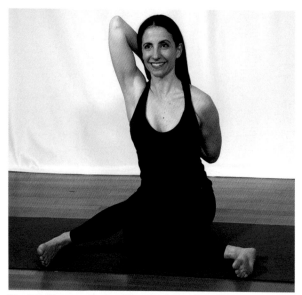

Fig. 9.8 Elbow supination: **Yoga Cow Face Pose (Gomukhasana)** (see Video 9.2 and Fig. 9.10).

maintaining an erect torso, place a cushion under your pelvis. Arms are by your sides with palms pressing into the floor.

- Engage your core, flex your knees, and slide your left foot under the right leg to place it outside of the right sitting bone. Then cross your right leg over the left, externally rotating the right hip to stack the right knee on top of the left; your right foot comes to the outside of the left sitting bone. Make sure to keep your ankles dorsiflexed and your pelvis neutral, with both sitting bones on the mat.
- Inhale and abduct your left arm to 90 degrees. Supinate your forearm and externally rotate your shoulder so that your palm faces the ceiling and perhaps toward the back of your mat (depending on your flexibility).
- On an exhale, continue abducting your left shoulder to 180 degrees and flex your left elbow to place your left hand as far down the midline of your back as possible; ideally, your left hand should rest around the level of your scapulae. Make sure that your spine remains neutral, with your chest broad and open, and scapulae depressing to create space between the shoulders and ears. Maintain this position of the left arm.
- Inhale and abduct your right arm to about 90 degrees. Exhale, pronate your right forearm, and internally

rotate your right shoulder so that your right palm faces the back of your mat and perhaps toward the ceiling (depending on your flexibility). Flex your right elbow and adduct your right shoulder to bring the dorsum of your hand as far up the midline of your back as possible. Ideally, your right forearm should be parallel with the vertical line of your spine and your right hand should rest around the level of your scapulae. Make sure that your spine remains neutral, with your chest broad and open, and scapulae depressing to create space between the shoulders and ears.

- Exhale and, if possible, clasp hands. If not possible, hold onto your shirt, a towel, or a yoga strap. Keep both elbows aligned toward the midline.
- Remain in this position for five slow breaths.
- On an exhale, release your arms, uncross your legs, and reverse sides.
- Ending position: On an exhale, release your arms back toward your sides. Unwind your legs and bring them into a cross-legged position.

PRONATION

Pitching a baseball, petting a dog, and performing a push-up are all activities that require pronation, a movement that, from the anatomical position, rotates the anterior forearm medially. Pronation is a very stable position for the forearm, with the radius firmly braced against the ulna. It occurs via mechanisms similar to those described for supination, in the reverse direction. The radius rotates around a stationary ulna bone at two joints: At the proximal radioulnar joint, the radial head spins within the radial notch of the ulna, and at the distal radioulnar joint, the ulnar notch of the radius rolls and slides on the head of the ulna. The direction in which the radius spins, rolls, and slides is medial—or, to the naked eye, the same direction as the moving thumb. Pronation is limited by the presence of supinator muscles and connective tissue structures at the ulnocarpal complex. (see Fig. 9.1). Try **Moving AnatoME** with **Yoga Cow Face Pose** (see Video 9.2). Note that your bottom forearm is pronated. If you are unable to hold hands, hold a towel or your shirt to maintain the connection between and proper positioning of your forearms.

Approximate Range of Motion

75 degrees (individuals who lack range may compensate by internally rotating at the shoulder)

Muscles and Innervation
See Fig. 9.9.

Muscle	Nerve
Pronator teres	Median n. (C6, C7)
Pronator quadratus	Anterior interosseous n. (C8, T1)
Flexor carpi radialis	Median n. (C6, C7)
Palmaris longus	Median n. (C7, C8)

Moving AnatoME Exercises
Elbow Pronation: Yoga Cow Face Pose
See Fig. 9.10, Video 9.2, and Box 9.2; see **Supination** for exercise steps.

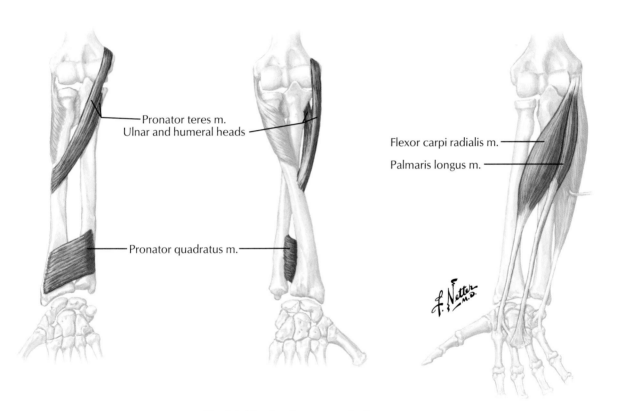

Pronator teres m.
Ulnar and humeral heads

Pronator quadratus m.

Flexor carpi radialis m.

Palmaris longus m.

Fig. 9.9 Muscles that pronate the forearm.

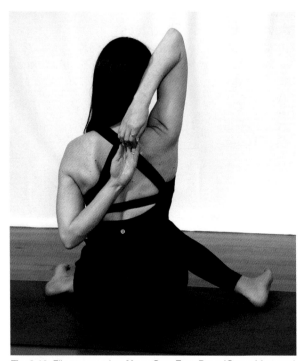

Fig. 9.10 Elbow pronation: **Yoga Cow Face Pose (Gomukhasana)** (see Video 9.2 and Fig. 9.8).

BOX 9.2   Together and Apart

Internal and external rotations of the arm are functionally linked to pronation and supination of the forearm, in order to allow the hand to rotate almost 360 degrees. Because of this intrinsic association, however, many individuals unwittingly internally rotate their shoulders when pronating their forearms, for example, when sitting at a desk typing at a computer. Try to break this pattern by keeping the shoulders in a neutral position and using your pronators—and not your internal rotators—to properly position your hands for typing.

10

Wrist

OVERVIEW

- The wrist is a compound joint that connects the forearm and hand.
- Articulations occur at the radius and carpal bones (the radiocarpal joint) and between the carpal bones (the midcarpal joints, intercarpal joints).
- Movements include flexion, extension, abduction, and adduction.
- Example exercises:
  - Flexion (**Yoga Hand-to-Foot Pose,** Video 10.1)
  - Extension (**Pilates Leg Pull Prep,** Video 10.2)
  - Abduction (**Wrist Strengthening Exercise,** Video 10.3)
  - Adduction (**Wrist Strengthening Exercise,** Video 10.3)

STRUCTURE AND FUNCTION

Although small in size, each wrist encompasses multiple complex articulations involving the distal radius, an articular disc at the distal ulna, and the eight carpal bones. Two articulations, the midcarpal and radiocarpal joints, play particularly important roles in allowing your hand to flex, extend, and move from side to side. Together, the joints act as a functional pair, allowing you to type, text, tie your shoes, and otherwise position your hand throughout the day (Fig. 10.1; see also Fig. 11.1).

The midcarpal joint is formed between the proximal and distal rows of carpal bones. These two rows are made up of eight irregularly shaped bones: The proximal row contains the scaphoid, lunate, triquetrum, and pisiform, and the distal row consists of the trapezium, trapezoid, capitate, and hamate (Clinical Focus 10.1). Many small intercarpal joints exist between these bones. Their movements are slight when compared with the midcarpal and radiocarpal joints, though integral to the full range of wrist motion. They also help absorb forces traveling from your hand to your forearm whether you are crawling, using crutches, or doing a handstand.

Moving proximally, the carpal bones articulate with the forearm at the radiocarpal joint. The joint's concave articulating surface is formed by the distal end of the radius and the articular disc overlying the distal end of the ulna; the joint's convex articulating surface includes the proximal borders of the scaphoid, lunate, and triquetrum. As with other synovial joints, the wrist joints contain a synovial membrane and a joint capsule strengthened by ligaments. Intercarpal ligaments, for example, help stabilize the connections between the carpal bones and safely transmit forces between the forearm and hand, so that the delicate wrist joints maintain their natural shape during movement.

The wrist is one of the most frequently manipulated joints in the body. Coordination between the radiocarpal and midcarpal joints allows you to flex, extend, abduct, and adduct your wrist multiple times per hour (see Fig. 10.2). Moving distally, the wrist joints coordinate with the carpometacarpal joints, which are formed by the distal carpal and proximal metacarpal bones, to further integrate movements of the hand (see Chapter 11, Hand).

MOVEMENT

To maneuver your hands in space, the wrist joint flexes, extends, abducts, and adducts (Fig. 10.2). The wrist can also circumduct, which is a combination of movements experienced when you circle your wrists. Each movement is enabled by the radiocarpal and midcarpal joints working in tandem, along with minor motion at the intercarpal

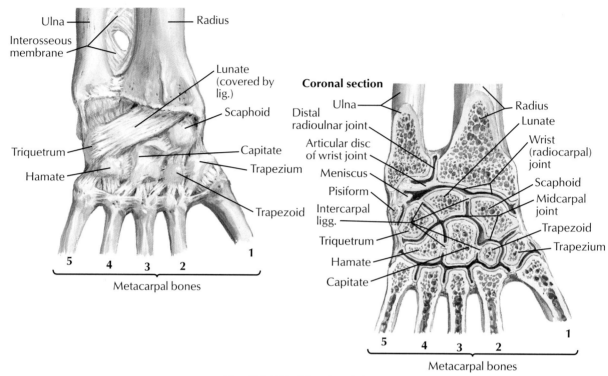

Fig. 10.1 Wrist joint: dorsal views.

joints. And although each movement can be isolated, the movements frequently occur together (eg, flexion with adduction). Moreover, wrist movements typically take place as part of a larger kinematic chain linking your forearms to your fingers. This is why an exercise instruction to "straighten your arms by your sides" assumes an equally straight wrist and hand (Practice What You Preach 10.1).

FLEXION

Rolling up your exercise mat requires repeated flexion at your wrist joints. It is a subtle movement that is deceivingly complex and not entirely understood. Current thinking indicates that wrist flexion occurs through longitudinal chains of joints that connect the wrist and hand, with primary importance placed on the middle chain. The middle chain, otherwise known as the central column, consists of articulations between the radius, lunate, capitate, and third metacarpal bone. The most proximal of the column's articulations (which include both the radiocarpal joint [at the radius and lunate] and the midcarpal joint [at the capitate and lunate]) move in tandem, as the surfaces

> ### PRACTICE WHAT YOU PREACH 10.1
> **Set Yourself Up for Success**
>
> When you were setting up your work-study area, how much attention did you pay to the height of your desk? Next time you are there, make sure you can place your wrists in a neutral position (neither flexed nor extended) to write or type. If needed, use cushions to prop yourself up on a chair, so you can bring your elbows level with your wrists; place books underneath your feet if they are dangling. If you're using a keyboard, consider ergonomic wrist guards or rests for further support. These small but effective modifications in your work-study posture will save your wrists from unwanted stress and any sequelae, such as carpal tunnel syndrome (see Clinical Focus 10.1; see also "Sitting Posture: Computer Desk Station" in Chapter 18).

of the involved bones roll and slide over each other. In wrist flexion, the midcarpal joint is the main actor.

The distal articulation of the central column is the carpometacarpal joint. Its rigid articulation between the capitate and third metacarpal bone allows the hand to

CLINICAL FOCUS 10.1 Carpal Tunnel Syndrome

Modern technology has both positive and negative effects, with carpal tunnel syndrome as an example of the latter. Often caused by repetitive wrist motions such as typing and texting, this common clinical syndrome involves the carpal tunnel, an area of the wrist formed by the eight carpal bones (the concave base of the tunnel) and the transverse carpal ligament (ie, the flexor retinaculum, the tunnel's overarching roof). The tunnel provides a passageway between the forearm and hand, encircling many structures such as tendons of the forearm flexor muscles (eg, flexor digitorum profundus and superficialis, flexor pollicus longus) and the median nerve. When inflamed, the tunnel may compress the median nerve, causing a peripheral neuropathy and forearm pain. In addition to repetitive motion, anything that decreases the size of the tunnel can cause symptoms, including inflammation due to diabetes, rheumatoid arthritis, or direct trauma (eg, a fall on an outstretched hand). Help prevent this condition by balancing wrist strength and flexibility. Exercises such as wrist circles or the **Yoga Hand-to-Foot Pose** (see Video 10.1) help to maintain supple wrists; light hand weights can also be used to gently build strength through range-of-motion exercises.

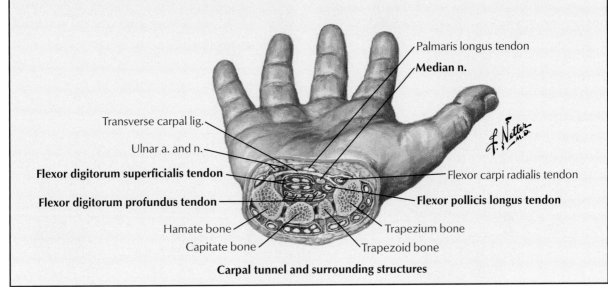

Carpal tunnel and surrounding structures

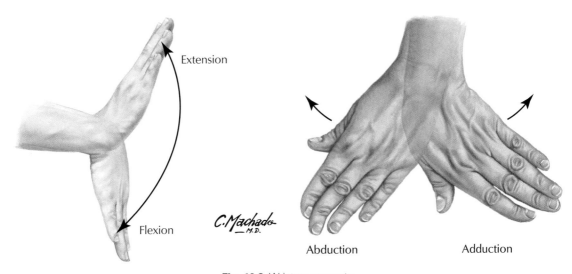

Fig. 10.2 Wrist movements.

follow the action of the wrist. In wrist flexion, then, this articulation brings the palm of the hand closer to the anterior surface of the forearm. As you can feel for yourself, wrist flexion is not an inherently stable position and is poorly suited to bear much body weight. As you try it, also observe how the flexion tends to be accompanied by a slight adduction. Try **Moving AnatoME** with the **Yoga Hand-to-Foot Pose** (Video 10.1) and experience a deep wrist flexion in addition to a stretch of your wrist extensors.

Approximate Range of Motion

70 degrees (at least 5 degrees is necessary to perform common personal care activities comfortably)

Muscles and Innervation

See Fig. 10.3.

Muscle	Nerve
Flexor carpi radialis	Median n. (C6, C7)
Flexor carpi ulnaris	Ulnar n. (C7, C8)
Palmaris longus	Median n. (C7, C8)
Flexor digitorum profundus	Medial portion, ulnar n. (C8, T1); lateral portion, median n. (C8, T1)
Flexor digitorum superficialis	Median n. (C7, C8, T1)
Flexor pollicis longus	Anterior interosseous n. (C8, T1)

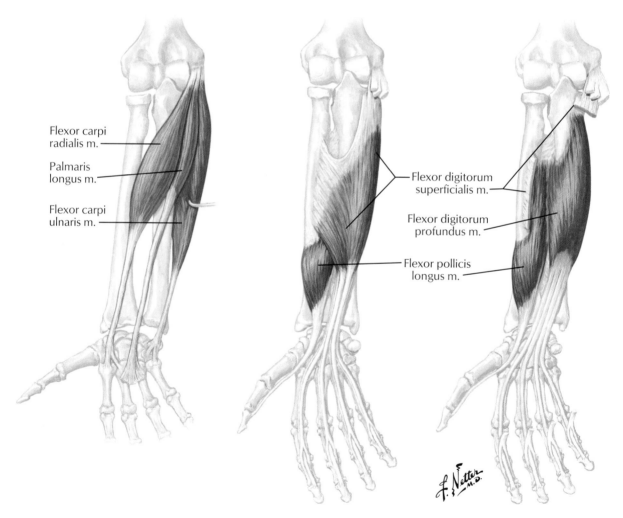

Flexor carpi radialis m.

Palmaris longus m.

Flexor carpi ulnaris m.

Flexor digitorum superficialis m.

Flexor digitorum profundus m.

Flexor pollicis longus m.

Fig. 10.3 Muscles that flex the wrist.

Moving AnatoME Exercise
Wrist Flexion: Yoga Hand-to-Foot Pose (Utthita Hasta Padangusthasana)

See Fig. 10.4 and Video 10.1.

- Starting position: Standing with your feet hip distance apart, in their natural parallel position. Weight is centered between both feet. Hands are resting on your waist.
- Engage your core, and on an exhale, flex forward at the hips, lowering your torso to the floor.
- Flex your knees and flex your wrists to place your palms under the soles of your feet; fingers point toward the heels.
- Extend your knees as much as possible (while maintaining the position of your hands under your feet) and relax into the pose, releasing any head and neck tension.
- Remain in this position for five rounds of breath.
- On the next inhale, place your hands back on your waist. Extend through the torso and return to a standing position.
- Ending position: Release your arms into a neutral stance.

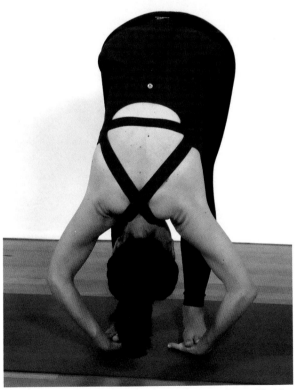

Fig. 10.4 Wrist flexion: **Yoga Hand-to-Foot Pose (Utthita Hasta Padangusthasana)** (see Video 10.1).

EXTENSION

As a baby, you crawled on your hands and knees, a form of locomotion necessitating extended wrists. Wrist extension functions like wrist flexion, but in the reverse direction. It is as poorly understood, and similarly involves the joints of the central column. The most proximal of these joints, the radiocarpal and midcarpal joints, move in tandem, as the surfaces of the involved bones (eg, radius, lunate, and capitate) roll and slide over each other; in wrist extension, the radiocarpal joint is the main actor. The distal articulation of the column, the carpometacarpal joint, is a rigid joint that allows the hand to follow the action of the wrist. During wrist extension, then, it brings the dorsum of the hand closer to the posterior surface of the forearm. Unlike wrist flexion, wrist extension is a stable position, as tension in the palmar capsule and surrounding ligaments and muscles stabilizes the joint. This stability is good for bearing and transferring weight, as when transferring from the floor to standing. See for yourself that extension is often accompanied by a slight abduction. Try **Moving AnatoME** with **Pilates Leg Pull Prep** (Video 10.2). Although it is a relatively stable position compared with flexion, wrist extension may feel uncomfortable if the muscles and ligaments around your wrist are weak and/or tight. You can place the base of your hands on a folded edge of your mat to decrease the amount of extension.

Approximate Range of Motion

60 degrees (at least 30 degrees is necessary to perform common personal care activities comfortably)

Muscles and Innervation

See Fig. 10.5.

Muscle	Nerve
Extensor carpi radialis longus	Radial n.(C6, C7)
Extensor carpi radialis brevis	Deep branch of radial n. (C7, C8)
Extensor carpi ulnaris	Radial n.(C6-C8)
Extensor digitorum	Posterior interosseous n. (C7, C8)
Extensor indices	Posterior interosseous nerve (C7, C8)
Extensor digiti minimi	Posterior interosseous nerve (C7, C8)
Extensor pollicis longus	Posterior interosseous nerve (C7, C8)

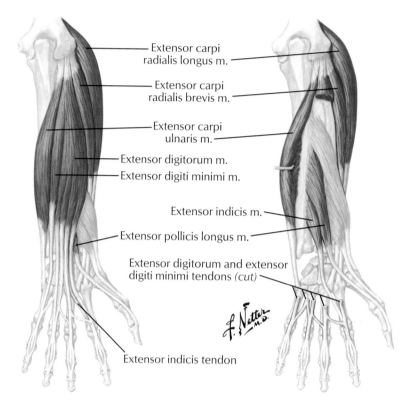

Extensor carpi
radialis longus m.

Extensor carpi
radialis brevis m.

Extensor carpi
ulnaris m.

Extensor digitorum m.

Extensor digiti minimi m.

Extensor indicis m.

Extensor pollicis longus m.

Extensor digitorum and extensor
digiti minimi tendons *(cut)*

Extensor indicis tendon

Fig. 10.5 Muscles that extend the wrist.

Moving AnatoME Exercise
Wrist Extension: Pilates Leg Pull Prep

See Fig. 10.6 and Video 10.2.

- Starting position: Similar to a quadruped position with hands underneath the shoulders and elbows extended, but in this position your knees should be a few inches behind the hips with your legs adducted and feet dorsiflexed. Press into the floor to mildly protract and stabilize the scapulae on the back. Your navel draws in to engage the lower abdominals, and your spine and pelvis are neutral.
- Inhale to prepare.
- Exhale and engage your core, adduct and activate your inner thighs, and press the bases of your toes into the floor as you slowly raise your knees 1 to 2 inches above the floor. Maintain a neutral spine.
- Inhale and slowly lower the knees back to the floor.
- Repeat six to eight times.
- Ending position: Lower your knees to the floor into a quadruped position.

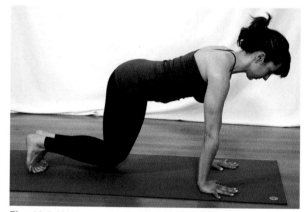

Fig. 10.6 Wrist extension: **Pilates Leg Pull Prep** (see Video 10.2).

ABDUCTION (RADIAL DEVIATION)

Wave goodbye in slow motion, as you would if you were sitting on a parade float. When the dorsal sides of your fingers point away from the midline, your wrist is in abduction (also called radial deviation). More complicated than flexion, the basic mechanism is nonetheless the same: synchronous rolls and slides at both the radiocarpal and midcarpal joints, with the midcarpal joint as the main mover. In radial deviation, most of the motion results from the midcarpal joint, with the carpometacarpal joint allowing the hand to follow the motion of the wrist. The resulting movement decreases the angle between the thumb and the lateral forearm. The range of radial deviation is less than that of ulnar deviation, limited by the ulnar collateral ligament and the carpal bones abutting against the styloid process of the radius. Try **Moving AnatoME** with **Wrist Strengthening Exercise** (Video 10.3). Isolate abduction by starting with your forearm parallel to the ground and wrist neutral. Abduction is the movement you employ to unscrew the lid from a jar (twisting it counterclockwise).

Approximate Range of Motion

60 degrees (at least 10 degrees is necessary to comfortably perform common personal care activities)

Muscles and Innervation

See Fig. 10.7.

Muscle	Nerve
Extensor carpi radialis longus	Radial n. (C6, C7)
Extensor carpi radialis brevis	Deep branch of radial n. (C7, C8)
Extensor pollicis longus	Posterior interosseous n. (C7, C8)
Extensor pollicis brevis	Posterior interosseous n. (C7, C8)
Flexor carpi radialis	Median n. (C6, C7)
Flexor pollicis longus	Anterior interosseous n. (C8, T1)
Abductor pollicis longus	Posterior interosseous n. (C7, C8)

Moving AnatoME Exercise

Wrist Abduction: Wrist Strengthening Exercise
See Fig. 10.8 and Video 10.3.

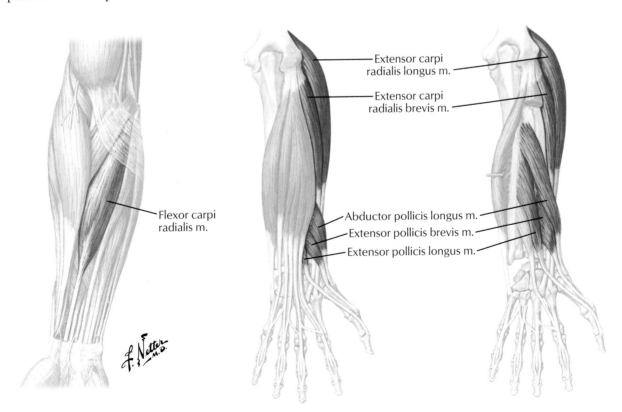

Flexor carpi radialis m.

Extensor carpi radialis longus m.

Extensor carpi radialis brevis m.

Abductor pollicis longus m.

Extensor pollicis brevis m.

Extensor pollicis longus m.

Fig. 10.7 Muscles that abduct the wrist. (*Muscle not shown*: flexor pollicis longus.)

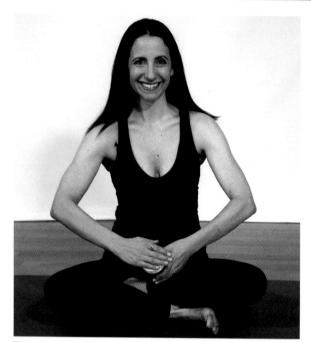

Fig. 10.8 Wrist abduction: **Wrist Strengthening Exercise** (see Video 10.3).

- Starting position: Obtain a twist-top jar (preferably one with a lid size that can you easily grasp in the palm of your hand), and sit in a comfortable position, either on a chair or cross-legged on the floor. Sit atop both sitting bones with a neutral spine.
- Hold the jar in your left hand. Flex your right elbow to 90 degrees and keep your right wrist in a neutral position so it is in the same plane as the forearm; keep the right arm adducted by your side.
- Isolate abduction of the right wrist as you twist the lid of the jar counterclockwise (off). Execute the movement from your wrist only, and do not incorporate shoulder adduction/abduction or internal/external rotation.
- Isolate adduction of the right wrist as you twist the lid of the jar clockwise (on). Execute the movement from your wrist only and do not incorporate shoulder adduction/abduction or internal/external rotation.
- Repeat the on-off cycle two to three times, and then switch to the left side.
- Ending position: Put the jar down, shake out your wrists, and relax your arms by your sides.

ADDUCTION (ULNAR DEVIATION)

In the anatomical position, the hands hang in a naturally adducted position, noticeable as a slight decrease in the angle between the pinky finger and medial forearm. Also called ulnar deviation, this movement parallels radial deviation; it is a poorly understood process combining rolls and slides at both the radiocarpal and midcarpal joints. In this instance, the radiocarpal joint is the main mover. Together with the rigid carpometacarpal joint, which allows the hand to follow the motion of the wrist, the resulting movement of the joints decreases the angle between the pinky and ulna. In general, the amount of adduction available is greater than abduction. Try **Moving AnatoME** with **Wrist Strengthening Exercise** (see Video 10.3). Isolate adduction by starting with your forearm parallel to the ground and wrist neutral. Adduction is the movement you employ to screw the lid onto a jar (twisting it clockwise).

Approximate Range of Motion

60 degrees (at least 15 degrees is necessary to perform common personal care activities comfortably)

Muscles and Innervation

See Fig. 10.9.

Muscle	Nerve
Extensor carpi ulnaris	Radial n. (C6-C8)
Flexor carpi ulnaris	Ulnar n. (C7, C8)

Moving AnatoME Exercise

Wrist Adduction: Wrist Strengthening Exercise
See Fig. 10.10 and Video 10.3; see **Abduction** for exercise steps.

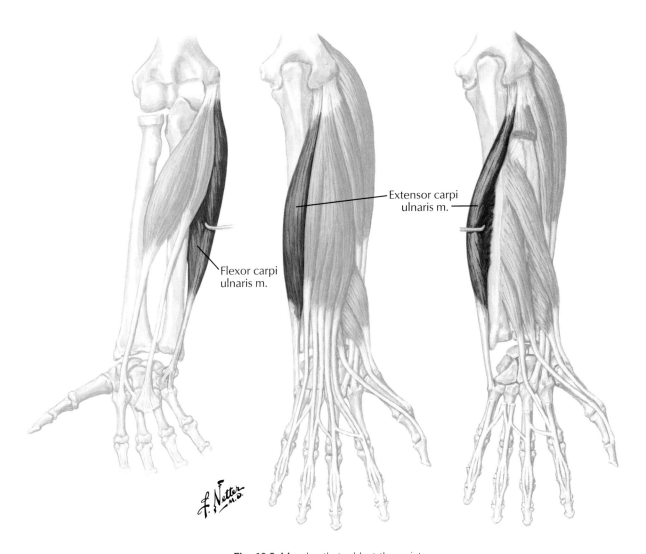

Extensor carpi
ulnaris m.

Flexor carpi
ulnaris m.

Fig. 10.9 Muscles that adduct the wrist.

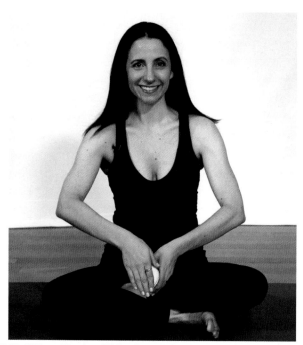

Fig. 10.10 Wrist adduction: **Wrist Strengthening Exercise** (see Video 10.3).

11

Hand

OVERVIEW

- The hand is the region distal to the forearm. It is composed of three regions: the carpus (wrist), metacarpus (palm), and digits (fingers).
- Articulations occur between the carpal bones (the intercarpal joints), carpal and metacarpal bones (the carpometacarpal joints), metacarpal bones and phalanges (the metacarpophalangeal joints), and phalanges (the interphalangeal joints). See Chapter 10 for articulations of the wrist (the radiocarpal, midcarpal joints).
- Movements include:
  - **Wrist:** flexion, extension, abduction, and adduction (see Chapter 10).
  - **Fingers:** flexion, extension, abduction, adduction, opposition, and reposition.
- Example exercises:
  - Finger flexion (**Yoga Wide-Legged Forward Bend,** Video 11.1)
  - Finger extension (**Pilates Leg Pull Prep,** see Video 10.2)
  - Finger abduction (**Yoga Downward-Facing Dog Pose,** Video 11.2)
  - Finger adduction (**Yoga Prayer Position,** Video 11.3)

STRUCTURE AND FUNCTION

Like the term *shoulder,* the term *hand* has many colloquial meanings (such as the hand you lend a friend. The physical hand has many regions, as well. Anatomically, the hand encompasses 27 major bones, plus 2 sesamoids. It is divided into three regions: the carpus (wrist), metacarpus (palm), and digits (fingers). Starting proximally, the wrist houses a complex of eight carpal bones with a multitude of joints, as detailed in Chapter 10, Wrist. In contrast, the metacarpus is a relatively simple region, consisting of five metacarpal bones (Greek *meta,* "after"; *carpus,* "wrist"). The five digits are the most distal members of the hand, made up of phalangeal bones. The second through fifth fingers each contain three phalanges: proximal, middle, and distal. The thumb, typically the shortest digit, contains only proximal and distal phalanges.

Interconnecting the hand's bones are an array of synovial joints, which fall into four categories: intercarpal, carpometacarpal, metacarpophalangeal, and interphalangeal. These joint names may seem complex, but they actually provide a useful guide for remembering the bones involved in the articulations (eg, the carpometacarpal joint occurs between the carpal and metacarpal bones) (Fig. 11.1).

Intercarpal Joints

The intercarpal (IC) joints occur between (Latin, *inter*) the carpal joints. Functionally, they interact with the forearm to position the hand in space, through small, gliding motions at the wrist, as discussed in Chapter 10, Wrist.

Carpometacarpal Joints

The carpometacarpal (CMC) joints connect the distal row of carpal bones with the bases of the five metacarpals (e.g. the third CMC joint is formed primarily between the capitate and the base of the third metacarpal). Together, the joints permit the palm to fit around many types of objects, as seen when one is holding a baseball;

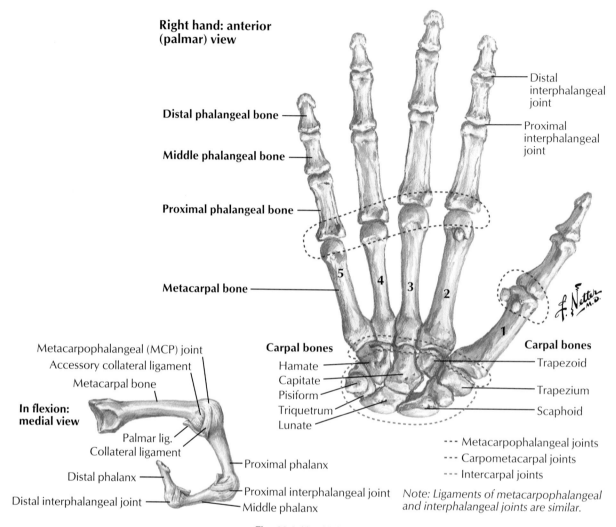

Right hand: anterior (palmar) view

Distal phalangeal bone

Middle phalangeal bone

Proximal phalangeal bone

Metacarpal bone

Distal interphalangeal joint

Proximal interphalangeal joint

Metacarpophalangeal (MCP) joint
Accessory collateral ligament
Metacarpal bone

In flexion: medial view

Palmar lig.
Collateral ligament
Distal phalanx
Distal interphalangeal joint

Proximal phalanx
Proximal interphalangeal joint
Middle phalanx

Carpal bones
Hamate
Capitate
Pisiform
Triquetrum
Lunate

Carpal bones
Trapezoid
Trapezium
Scaphoid

- - - Metacarpophalangeal joints
- - - Carpometacarpal joints
- - - Intercarpal joints

Note: Ligaments of metacarpophalangeal and interphalangeal joints are similar.

Fig. 11.1 Hand joints.

the joints also link motions of the wrist to motions of the rest of the hand and the fingers, as seen when one is throwing a baseball. Of note, the CMC joints between the carpal bones and metacarpals 2 through 5 permit relatively limited gliding movements; the joints at digits 2 through 3 exhibit little movement as they are also used for stability of the hand, with slightly more movement available at digits 4 and 5. In contrast, the saddle-shaped CMC joint between the first metacarpal and trapezium enables a much broader range of motion, which is part of the defining mobility of the human thumb. Wiggle

your fingers to see for yourself that your thumb can move through a wider range of motion.

Metacarpophalangeal Joints

The metacarpophalangeal (MCP) joints connect the metacarpals to the phalanges. Stability at these joints is integral to support of the arches of the hand. In terms of mobility, these joints allow flexion and extension of the proximal phalanges, as well as abduction, adduction, circumduction, and small amounts of rotation. Like the CMC joints, the MCP joints of the second through fifth fingers increase in range medially. Test this for yourself by making a fist and noting the increased flexion of the medial digits.

Interphalangeal Joints

The interphalangeal (IP) joints occur between the distal, middle, and proximal phalanges. In the fingers, the proximal IP joints are formed by the heads of the proximal phalanges and the bases of the middle phalanges; the distal IP joints are formed by the heads of the middle phalanges and the bases of the distal phalanges. The thumb has only two phalanges and therefore one IP joint. These joints allow for flexion and extension of the small bones that form your fingers.

Although relatively small, each of these joints functions like the larger synovial joints in the body (eg, hip and elbow) and likewise contains its own synovial membranes, capsule, and ligaments. Together, they allow your hand to grasp, pinch, and otherwise form positions that allow you to hold a hammer, open a door, flip pages, and write notes. Thanks to your bipedal stance, your hands are able to interface with your environment by both sensing it (eg, feeling the doorknob) and acting upon it (eg, turning it). Plus, they provide important tools for nonverbal communication, as they express thoughts and emotions through gestures (eg, a clenched fist expresses anger) and art. Your hands, of course, do not act alone; rather, they are the distal end of the upper extremity's kinetic chain, which starts at the shoulder complex. The wide range of motion available through the shoulder joints, then, is not just for movement of your arms, but it is also for movement and positioning of your hands. See for yourself, as you use your hand to grab an item in front of you; you need to protract your scapula, flex your arm, extend your elbow—and more—for your hand to do its job (Practice What You Preach 11.1).

MOVEMENT

Wiggle your fingers to appreciate the dexterity that allows you to hold a spoon or type texts. These daily activities occur by virtue of movements at the joints of the hand (IC, CMC, MCP, and IP). As discussed in Chapter 10, Wrist, the IC joints, along with the radiocarpal and midcarpal joints, position the hand in space by flexing, extending, and deviating it medially and laterally. The intrinsic hand joints, specifically the MCP and IP joints, fine-tune the movements by permitting flexion, extension, abduction, and adduction, plus small amounts of rotation of our fingers (Fig. 11.2). The thumb can also oppose, a movement of central importance to human dexterity. *Opposition* is a special term that describes the movement of the thumb across the palm to contact the tips of the other fingers. Its motion results from a complex interaction featuring the CMC joint of the thumb working in concert with other joints of the hand (depending on which finger the thumb is opposing). *Reposition*, in contrast, is the term that describes the movement that returns an opposed thumb to anatomical position (Box 11.1).

As with other joints, the range of motion of the hand joints is determined by muscular attachments, the shape and orientation of the articulations of the bones, and the presence or absence of collateral ligaments. As a defining feature, however, hand range of motion also strongly depends upon the positioning of neighboring joints. For instance, keep your wrist neutral and make a fist. Now, relax your hand, flex your wrist, and see how far you can flex your fingers into your palm. It's likely that flexion will be more limited. This restricted range of motion occurs because the tendons of the forearm flexors and extensors are not long enough to allow a maximal range of motion at the wrist and fingers simultaneously (recall that the muscle tendons responsible for hand movements come from not only the hand itself, but also the forearm).

Finger movements

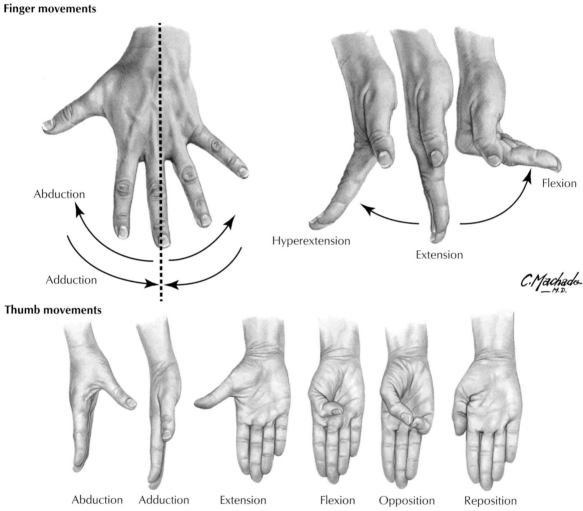

Thumb movements

Abduction   Adduction   Extension   Flexion   Opposition   Reposition

Fig. 11.2 Finger and thumb movements.

Finger dexterity, inclusive of thumb opposability, is a defining feature of human life, with its utility culminating in your ability to grip, grasp, or otherwise take hold of an object. The act of taking hold of something, known as prehension, has allowed humankind to manipulate (Latin *manus*, "hand") the environment as no other animal can. Throughout time, our ability to craft tools, light fires, and more has lifted *Homo sapiens* to the top of the evolutionary chain. Our prehensile activities can be classified in two main forms: a grip (or grasp) and a pinch. Activities in these two groups can be further delineated into power and precision categories; a power grip, for example, helps you hold a hammer, whereas a precision pinch helps you hold a pen. So the next time you grab a cup of coffee or hold the door open for a friend, take a moment to take hold (literally) of the evolutionary refinement of your hands.

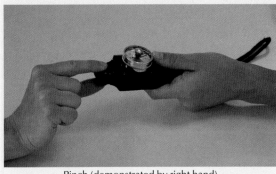

Pinch (demonstrated by right hand)

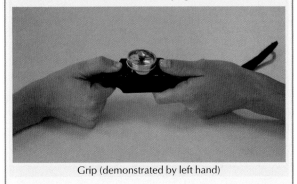

Grip (demonstrated by left hand)

FLEXION

When you hold a pen to take notes, you flex your fingers. In this position, all five digits flex at the MCP and IP joints, with limited motion also occurring at the CMC joints. For digits 2 to 5, this flexion occurs in the sagittal plane about a medial-lateral axis of rotation; the amount of movement increases from the second to the fifth digit. Flexion brings the palmar aspects of these fingers closer to the anterior surface of the forearm. In contrast, and due to the positioning of the first metacarpal, the thumb flexes in the frontal plane. This positioning allows it to intersect with the other fingers in flexion to enable prehensility (eg, gripping and pinching) versus parallel movement. Because the thumb is rotated almost 90 degrees in relation to the other fingers, flexion brings its palmar surface across the palm. The thumb's flexion is also notable for a greater range of motion, thanks to additional mobility at the first CMC joint. Try **Moving AnatoME** with **Yoga Wide-Legged Forward Bend** (see Video 11.1) with your arms extended overhead and hands clasped. Flex your fingers to seal the palms of the hands together, noting how that grip facilitates a full activation of the upper extremity and a greater stretch through the shoulder.

Approximate Range of Motion

Finger: MCP, 100 degrees; PIP (proximal interphalangeal), 120 degrees; DIP (distal interphalangeal), 90 degrees
Thumb: CMC, 50 degrees; MCP, 60 degrees; IP, 70 degrees

Muscles and Innervation

See Fig. 11.3.

Muscle	Nerve
Fingers	
Flexor digiti minimi	Deep branch of ulnar n. (C8, T1)
Flexor digitorum profundus	Median portion: ulnar n. (C8, T1); Lateral portion: median n. (C8, T1)
Flexor digitorum superficialis	Median n. (C7-T1)
Lumbricals	Lateral: median n. (C8, T1); Medial: deep branch of ulnar n. (C8, T1)
Thumb	
Flexor pollicis brevis	Median n. (C8, T1)
Flexor pollicis longus	Anterior interosseous n. (C8, T1)
Abductor pollicis brevis	Median n. (C8, T1)
Adductor pollicis	Deep branch of ulnar n. (C8, T1)

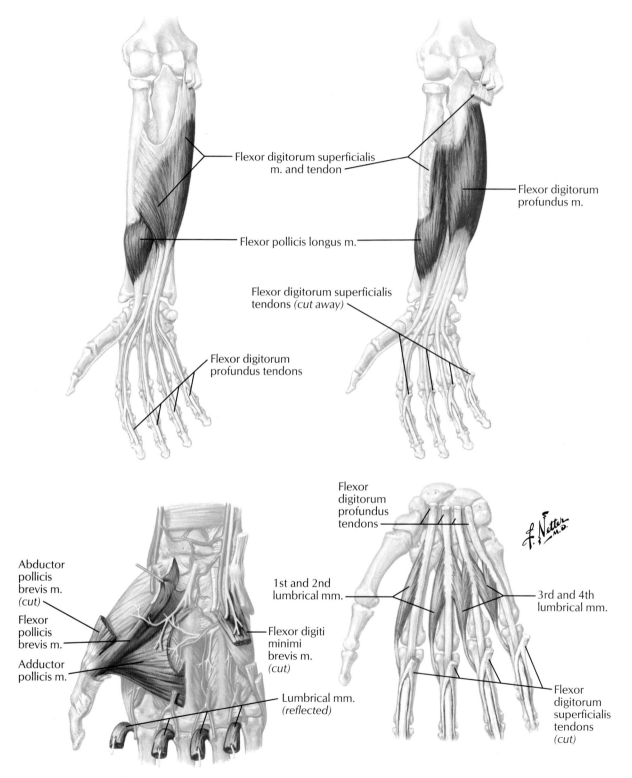

Flexor digitorum superficialis m. and tendon

Flexor digitorum profundus m.

Flexor pollicis longus m.

Flexor digitorum superficialis tendons *(cut away)*

Flexor digitorum profundus tendons

Flexor digitorum profundus tendons

Abductor pollicis brevis m. *(cut)*

Flexor pollicis brevis m.

Adductor pollicis m.

1st and 2nd lumbrical mm.

3rd and 4th lumbrical mm.

Flexor digiti minimi brevis m. *(cut)*

Lumbrical mm. *(reflected)*

Flexor digitorum superficialis tendons *(cut)*

Fig. 11.3 Muscles that flex the fingers. *(Muscle not shown:* flexor pollicis longus.)

Moving AnatoME Exercise

Finger Flexion: Yoga Wide-Legged Forward Bend (Prasarita Padottanasana C)

 See Fig. 11.4 and Video 11.1 .

- Starting position: Standing with your feet hip distance apart in their natural parallel position. Weight is centered between both feet. Hands are on your waist.
- Step your feet 3 to 4 feet apart. Clasp your palms together behind your back, flexing your fingers to interlace them.
- Inhale and lengthen your torso. On the exhale, engage your core and flex forward at the hips, lowering your torso to the floor. Extend your arms so that your hands reach toward the floor.
- Keep your torso long, head relaxed, and hands reaching toward the floor. Breathe for five cycles.
- On an inhale, lift your torso back to a standing position and lower your arms in tandem.
- Ending position: Unclasp your palms, releasing your hands by your sides, and step your feet together.

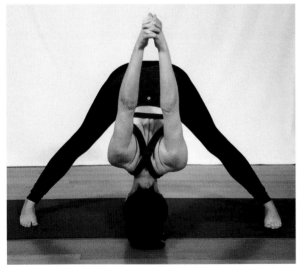

Fig. 11.4 Finger flexion: **Yoga Wide-Legged Forward Bend (Prasarita Padottanasana C)** (see Video 11.1).

EXTENSION

When you push your office door shut, you extend your hand and fingers. In this position, all five digits extend at the MCP and IP joints. Extension brings the dorsum of these fingers closer to the posterior surface of the forearm. Extension works like flexion: for digits 2 to 5 at the MCP and IP joints, extension occurs in the sagittal plane about a medial-lateral axis of rotation, with greater mobility allowed at the more medial joints. In contrast, and because of the positioning of the first metacarpal, the thumb extends in the frontal plane, with the help of the CMC joint. Because the thumb is rotated almost 90 degrees in relation to the other fingers, extension is the movement that returns the thumb to its anatomical position (try it for yourself). The thumb's extension is more limited than its flexion, as it is nearly fully extended at the CMC joint in anatomical position. Try **Moving AnatoME** with **Pilates Leg Pull Prep** (see Video 10.2). Engage your hand and finger extensors to help you isometrically push into the floor and form a solid foundation. You may even feel some relief from pressure in your shoulders.

Approximate Range of Motion

Finger: MCP, 45 degrees; PIP, 0 degrees; DIP, minimal
Thumb: CMC, 15 degrees; MCP, negligible; IP, 20 degrees

Muscles and Innervation

See Fig. 11.5 (see Fig. 11.3 for lumbricals).

Muscle	Nerve
Fingers	
Extensor digiti minimi	Posterior interosseous n. (C7, C8)
Extensor indices	Posterior interosseous n. (C7, C8)
Lumbricals	Lateral: median n. (C8, T1); Medial:deep branch of ulnar n. (C8, T1)
Thumb	
Extensor pollicis brevis	Posterior interosseous n.
Extensor pollicis longus	(C7, C8)
Abductor pollicis longus	

Moving AnatoME Exercise

Finger Extension: Pilates Leg Pull Prep

See Fig. 10.4, Video 10.2 , and Clinical Focus 11.1.

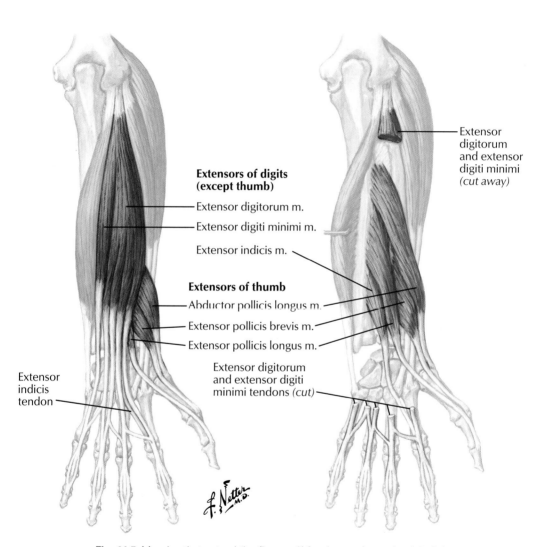

**Extensors of digits
(except thumb)**

Extensor digitorum m.

Extensor digiti minimi m.

Extensor indicis m.

Extensors of thumb

Abductor pollicis longus m.

Extensor pollicis brevis m.

Extensor pollicis longus m.

Extensor digitorum
and extensor digiti
minimi tendons *(cut)*

Extensor
indicis
tendon

Extensor
digitorum
and extensor
digiti minimi
(cut away)

Fig. 11.5 Muscles that extend the fingers. (*Muscle not shown:* lumbricals.)

CLINICAL FOCUS 11.1   Rheumatoid Arthritis

Rheumatoid arthritis (RA) is a disorder that can cause devastating destruction of the body's joints (as well as organs). Unlike osteoarthritis, which is a degenerative disorder, RA is an autoimmune disease, launched by the body's own disease-fighting system. The initial target of the immune attack on a joint is the synovial tissue, which fills with inflammatory cells and noxious by-products. The diseased synovial tissue swells and protrudes into the joint, inciting further inflammation and eventual degradation of the cartilage and bone; tendons and other musculoskeletal components may also be affected. RA typically affects the hands (and feet) first, with a marked impact in the form of ulnar deviation, boutonniere deformity, and/or swan-neck deformity. Although remissions occur and medical therapies can help manage the disease, RA is typically considered incurable. To ease the effects of RA in the hands, rehabilitation may focus on improving strength and/or flexibility with focused exercises, for example, hand and finger extension held for 5 to 10 seconds. Patient education to reduce unnecessary joint stress also helps (eg, replacing doorknobs with handles), as do at-home pain management techniques such as the deep breathing technique of **Alternate Nostril Breathing (Anuloma Viloma)** shown in Video 18.5 .

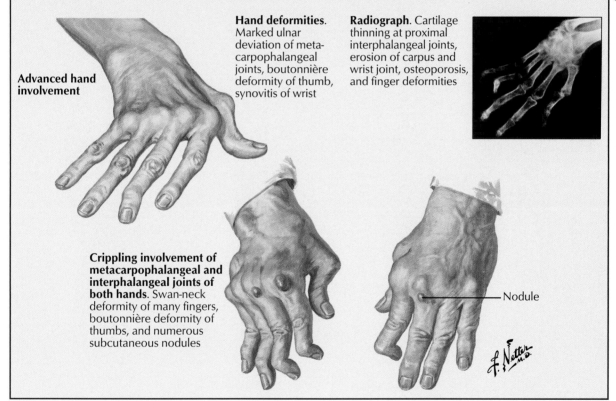

Advanced hand involvement

Hand deformities. Marked ulnar deviation of meta-carpophalangeal joints, boutonnière deformity of thumb, synovitis of wrist

Radiograph. Cartilage thinning at proximal interphalangeal joints, erosion of carpus and wrist joint, osteoporosis, and finger deformities

Crippling involvement of metacarpophalangeal and interphalangeal joints of both hands. Swan-neck deformity of many fingers, boutonnière deformity of thumbs, and numerous subcutaneous nodules

—Nodule

ABDUCTION

To display the number 5 with your hand, you abduct your fingers. In this action, the middle finger becomes the midline from which the other phalanges move away (while the middle finger's movement can be referenced as either radial or ulnar). Occurring primarily at the MCP joints, abduction occurs for fingers 2 to 5 in the frontal plane about an anterior-posterior axis of rotation. See for yourself that it is a much easier movement to facilitate with the MCPs in extension than flexion; also, that mobility is greatest in the second and fifth digits (as there are no adjacent digits to limit motion). For the thumb, abduction occurs in the sagittal plane; motion is greatest at the CMC joint and considered accessory at the MCP joint. Abduction is the forward movement of the thumb, away from the palm of the hand. Try **Moving AnatoME** with **Yoga Downward-Facing Dog Pose** (Video 11.2). Take time to properly position your hand with all five fingers active and abducted. Note how this hand positioning facilitates a wider foundation and greater stability through the rest of your upper extremity.

Approximate Range of Motion

Finger: MCP, 20 degrees
Thumb: CMC, 45 degrees

Muscles and Innervation

See Fig. 11.6.

Muscle	Nerve
Fingers	
Abductor digiti minimi	Deep branch of ulnar
Dorsal interossei	n. (C8, T1)
Thumb	
Abductor pollicis brevis	Median n. (C8, T1)
Abductor pollicis longus	Posterior interosseous
	n. (C7, C8)

Moving AnatoME Exercise

Finger Abduction: Yoga Downward-Facing Dog Pose (Adho Mukha Svanasana)

See Fig. 11.7 and Video 11.2.

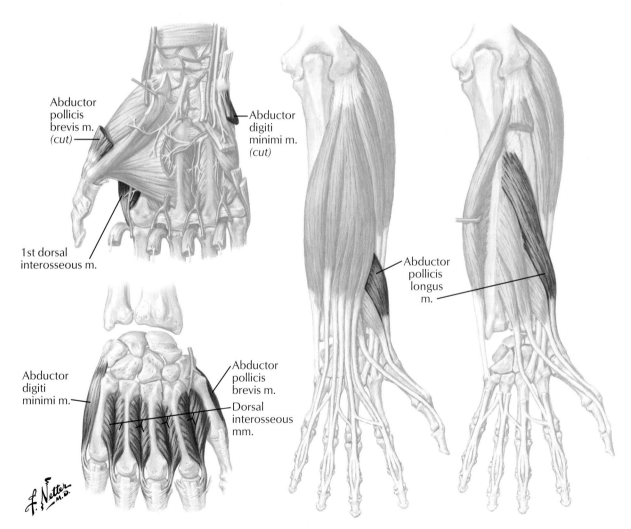

Fig. 11.6 Muscles that abduct the fingers.

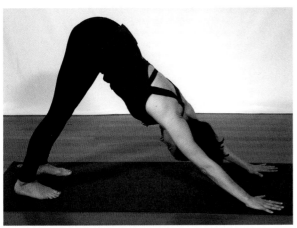

Fig. 11.7 Finger abduction: **Yoga Downward-Facing Dog Pose (Adho Mukha Svanasana)** (see Video 11.2).

- Starting position: In a quadruped position on your hands and knees, with wrists under shoulders and knees under hips. The heels are dorsiflexed and toes are extended and curled under. Your torso is parallel to the floor, and your neck is neutral, with the gaze down and slightly in front of you.
- Exhale, press your palms into the floor, and extend your knees. Feel your sitting bones lift toward the ceiling. Reach your heels toward the floor, even if they do not touch it. If needed, keep a soft bend in your knees.
- As you press your hands into the floor, abduct your fingers to create a stable foundation. Stabilize your scapulae on your back. Your head and neck should remain in line with your spine, with your gaze toward your feet.
- Remain here for five rounds of breath.
- Ending position: Flex your knees and lower them to the floor, returning to a quadruped position.

ADDUCTION

To give a "high five," you adduct your fingers. In this action, the middle finger becomes the midline toward which the other fingers move. Like abduction, adduction originates at the MCP joints, occurring for fingers 2 to 5 in the frontal plane about an anterior-posterior axis of rotation. For the thumb, adduction occurs in the sagittal plane; motion is minimal at the MCP joint and greatest at the CMC joint. Adduction describes the movement that returns the thumb to the plane of the hand. Try **Moving AnatoME** with **Yoga Prayer Position** (Video 11.3). Invoked in many cultures, this well-recognized hand position often connotes reverence or gratitude. In yoga class, you may encounter it before, between, or after poses to help you (re)center.

Approximate Range of Motion

Finger: 0 degrees
Thumb: 30 degrees

Muscles and Innervation

See Fig. 11.8.

Muscle	Nerve
Fingers	
Palmar interossei	Deep branch of ulnar n. (C8, T1)
Thumb	
Adductor pollicis	Deep branch of ulnar n. (C8, T1)

Moving AnatoME Exercise

Finger Adduction: Yoga Prayer Position (Anjali Mudra)
See Fig. 11.9 and Video 11.3 .

- Starting position: Standing with your feet hip distance apart, in their natural parallel position. Weight is centered between both feet. Arms relax by your sides.
- Form a firm foundation by isometrically extending and spreading your toes evenly along the floor. Lift the arches of both feet, and press your feet into the floor as you isometrically engage the muscles of your thighs and legs, rotating your thighs slightly inward.
- Lengthen your sitting bones toward the floor while elongating through your head and neck.
- Inhale and bring your palms together in front of your chest. Your fingers are adducted; thumbs may lightly touch your sternum. Elbows point toward the floor.
- Press your palms evenly against each other and nod your head slightly toward them. Keep your chest open and broad.
- Remain here for five rounds of breath.
- Ending position: Inhale and lift your head. Exhale, lower your arms, and return to a neutral stance.

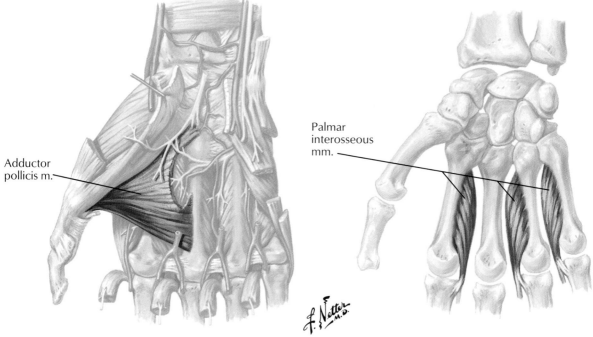

Adductor pollicis m.

Palmar interosseous mm.

Fig. 11.8 Muscles that adduct the fingers.

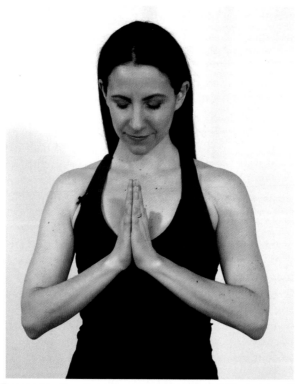

Fig. 11.9 Finger adduction: **Yoga Prayer Position (Anjali Mudra)** (see Video 11.3).

12

Regional Overview of Lower Extremity

The lower limbs reach from the ilia of the pelvis to the most distal tips of the toes. These two extremities not only support your body's weight but also move your body around on two feet, with an efficient expenditure of energy. Bipedalism, the ability to ambulate on two feet, evolved over millions of years, and it is part of what distinguishes our *Homo sapiens* species from most of the animal kingdom. Upright locomotion and posture are key elements of the human body; their evolution has freed up our hands for eating, building, shopping, and otherwise interacting with the world. This is in contrast to animals that need all four extremities for locomotion, and use them primarily for that purpose, as do dogs, cats, cows, and other quadrupeds.

The lower extremity is divided into discrete regions (Fig. 12.1):
- The **pelvic region** houses the pelvis, a bony basin that provides a biomechanical junction between the axial skeleton and lower extremities. It articulates with the trunk at the sacroiliac joints and connects to the lower limbs at the hip joints.
- The **gluteal region** is positioned posterolaterally on the body, between the iliac crests and gluteal folds (creases of skin delineating the bottom of the buttocks).
- The **thigh** runs, anteriorly, between the inguinal ligament and the knee and, posteriorly, between the gluteal fold and the knee.
- The **leg** extends from the knee to the ankle.
- The **foot** comprises all of the anatomy distal to the ankle.

BONES OF THE LOWER EXTREMITY

The skeletal framework of the lower extremity supports bipedalism and includes the following bones (Fig. 12.2):
- **Pelvic region**: Ischium, ilium, pubis
- **Thigh**: Femur
- **Leg**: Tibia, fibula, patella
- **Foot:**
  - **Tarsal bones:** (Proximal row) talus and calcaneus; (intermediate row) navicular; (distal row) cuboid and lateral, intermediate, and medial cuneiforms
  - **Metatarsal bones:** Metatarsals I, II, III, IV, V (medial to lateral)
  - **Phalanges:** Proximal (toes I to V), middle (toes II to V), distal (toes I to V)

MUSCLES OF THE LOWER EXTREMITY

The muscles that move the lower extremities primarily arise from lower extremity regions, including gluteal, thigh, leg, and foot (Tables 12.1 to 12.3 and Figs. 12.3 to 12.5). Additional muscle groups related to the lower extremity are discussed in axial skeleton (Chapters 4 to 6). One example is the iliopsoas, a posterior abdominal wall muscle, which exerts its major force at the hip joint but, due to its location, is included in Chapter 4, Regional Overview of Axial Skeleton. A second example includes the pelvic diaphragm muscles, which are located in the pelvic region, but due to their role in the core are discussed in Chapter 6, under "Movement: The Core" (Box 12.1).

Anterior view   **Posterior view**

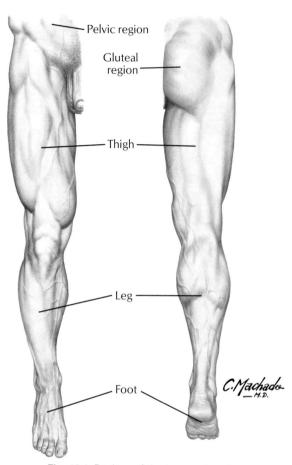

Fig. 12.1 Regions of the lower extremity.

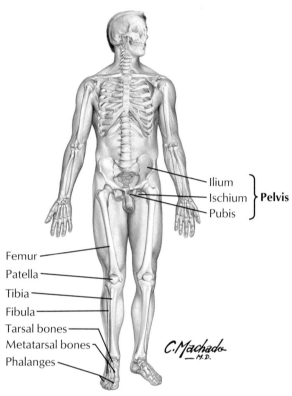

Fig. 12.2 Bones of the lower extremity.

Despite their various locations in the lower limb, all of the muscles that move the extremity are designed and compartmentalized to efficiently walk, hop, skip, and jump the body through space—types of locomotion that are contingent on an erect posture. Surprisingly, many of the muscles responsible for our bipedalism are similar to muscles that were long ago responsible for our forerunners' quadrupedalism. One exception is the human gluteus maximus muscle. With greater power, a "new" position in the body, and a big role in stabilization, the gluteus maximus has been shaped throughout evolution to permit our current upright lifestyle.

TABLE 12.1 Muscles and Muscle Compartments of the Gluteal Region and Thigh (See Fig. 12.3)

Muscles and Compartments	Notes
Gluteal Region **Superficial:** Gluteus maximus, gluteus medius, gluteus minimus, tensor fasciae latae **Deep**: Piriformis, gemellus superior, gemellus inferior, obturator internus, obturator externus, quadratus femoris	The superficial muscles are relatively large and play an active role in hip extension and abduction. The deep muscles are much smaller and collectively known as the deep lateral rotators for the primary movement they enable at the hip.
Thigh **Anterior:** Sartorius, quadriceps femoris: rectus femoris, vastus lateralis, vastus medialis, vastus intermedius **Posterior:** Hamstrings: semitendinosus, semimembranosus, biceps femoris **Medial:** Adductor longus, adductor brevis, adductor magnus, gracilis, pectineus	As a rule, the anterior muscles enable hip flexion and knee extension; the posterior muscles enable hip extension and knee flexion, and the medial muscles are hip adductors. Note that the body's strongest hip flexor is the combined iliopsoas muscle, located in the posterior abdominal wall.

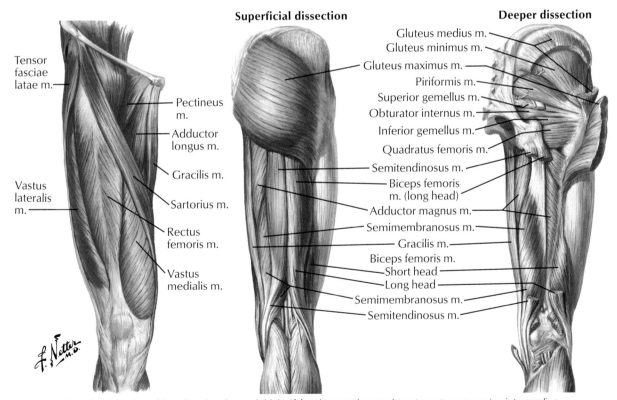

Fig. 12.3 Muscles of the gluteal region and thigh. (*Muscles not shown:* obturator externus, vastus intermedius, adductor brevis.)

TABLE 12.2	**Muscles and Muscle Compartments of the Leg (See** Fig. 12.4**)**
Muscles and Compartments	**Notes**
Anterior: Tibialis anterior, extensor digitorum longus, extensor hallucis longus, fibularis tertius	Most of the leg muscles cross the ankle joint to act on the foot. As a rule, the anterior muscles are dorsiflexors. The two lateral muscles evert the foot. The superficial and deep posterior muscles, although separated by a layer of deep fascia, function mainly to plantarflex the foot.
Lateral: Fibularis longus, fibularis brevis	
Posterior (superficial): Gastrocnemius, soleus, plantaris	
Posterior (deep): Tibialis posterior, flexor digitorum longus, flexor hallucis longus, popliteus	

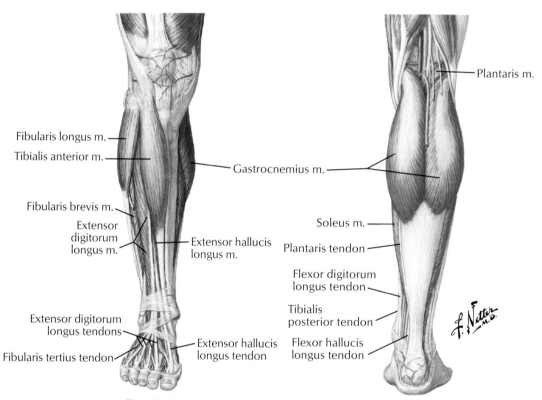

Plantaris m.

Fibularis longus m.

Tibialis anterior m.

Gastrocnemius m.

Fibularis brevis m.

Extensor digitorum longus m.

Extensor hallucis longus m.

Soleus m.

Plantaris tendon

Flexor digitorum longus tendon

Tibialis posterior tendon

Extensor digitorum longus tendons

Fibularis tertius tendon

Extensor hallucis longus tendon

Flexor hallucis longus tendon

Fig. 12.4 Muscles of the leg. (*Muscle not shown:* popliteus.)

TABLE 12.3	**Muscles and Muscle Compartments of the Foot (See** Fig. 12.5**)**
Muscles and Compartments	**Notes**
Dorsal: Extensor digitorum brevis **Plantar (first layer, most superficial):** Abductor hallucis, flexor digitorum brevis, abductor digiti minimi **Plantar (second layer):** Lumbricals, quadratus plantae **Plantar (third layer):** Adductor hallucis, flexor hallucis brevis, flexor digiti minimi brevis **Plantar (fourth layer, deepest):** Plantar interossei, dorsal interossei	The plantar muscle layers are arranged from superficial (first) to deep (fourth). Together with the single dorsal layer, the intrinsic muscles move the foot and toes. Recall that there are also extrinsic muscles arising from the leg that move these regions, too.

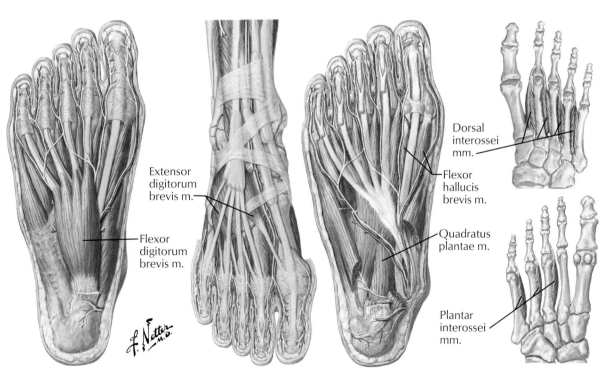

Extensor digitorum brevis m.

Flexor digitorum brevis m.

Dorsal interossei mm.

Flexor hallucis brevis m.

Quadratus plantae m.

Plantar interossei mm.

Fig. 12.5 Muscles of the foot. (*Muscle not shown:* adductor hallucis.)

13

Hip

OVERVIEW

- The hip is a multiaxial ball-and-socket joint that connects the pelvis and thigh.
- Its articulation occurs between the pelvis and femur (at the acetofemoral joint).
- Movements include flexion, extension, abduction, adduction, external rotation, internal rotation, and circumduction.
- Movements occur in two ways: femoral-on-pelvic and pelvic-on-femoral.
- Example exercises:
  - Flexion (**Yoga Tree Pose,** Video 13.1; **Pilates Pelvic Tilts,** Video 13.2)
  - Extension (**Pilates Swimming,** Video 13.3; **Pilates Pelvic Tilts,** Video 13.2)
  - Abduction (**Yoga Triangle Pose,** Video 13.5; **Pilates Side Leg Series (Abduction),** Video 13.4)
  - Adduction (**Yoga Triangle Pose,** Video 13.5; **Pilates Side Leg Series (Adduction),** Video 13.6)
  - External rotation (**Yoga Warrior II Pose,** Video 13.8; **Pilates Clamshell,** Video 13.7)
  - Internal rotation (**Yoga Warrior I Pose,** Video 13.9; **Pilates Clamshell,** Video 13.7)

STRUCTURE AND FUNCTION

Put your hands on your hips. Where are they? Many individuals will place their hands on their waists, or on the lateral aspects of their thighs, unaware that their hips are joints that are located deep within the groins.

The hip (acetabulofemoral joint) is a synovial ball-and-socket joint that connects the pelvic girdle to a lower extremity, with the femur as the "ball" and the acetabulum as the "socket." It exhibits the typical features of a synovial joint: articulating surfaces covered in hyaline cartilage, an inner synovial membrane that nourishes the joint surfaces and aids mobility, and a loose fibrous capsule encasing the joint. With the head of the femur almost entirely encompassed within the acetabulum, the hip is a deep joint, as well as one of the largest in the body (the knee is the largest) (Fig. 13.1 and Practice What You Preach 13.1).

The hip joint's depth and strength set it apart from the shoulder joint, which is also a ball-and-socket joint with a wide range of motion. For good reason, too: In tandem with the pelvic girdle, the hip not only bears the weight of the upper body but also transfers it to the lower limbs, whether you are standing or moving. Additional sources of stability include supporting structures like the labrum lining the acetabular rim and ligaments enveloping the joint. In fact, the iliofemoral ligament, a triangular-shaped band (with a Y appearance) connecting the ilium and femur, is considered to be one of the strongest ligaments in the body. Together with the ischiofemoral and pubofemoral ligaments, it not only stabilizes the joint but also increases its efficiency so you can stand for prolonged periods of time while using minimal muscular energy (Practice What You Preach 13.2).

The hip is an excellent stabilizer, designed to withstand large forces that can occur during walking and other activities. It mobilizes humans, as well. It allows for a full range of multiaxial motions of the thigh: flexion, extension, abduction, adduction, rotation, and circumduction (see Fig. 13.3). Hefty muscles such as the psoas and gluteus maximus act on the joint, with additional torque supplied by the surrounding ligaments. For instance, when you extend your hip quickly before flexing it to kick a soccer ball, this "wind-up" stores elastic energy (like a rubber band would) in the large ligaments. When you kick, this energy is released, amplifying the power of your hip flexor muscles (Fig. 13.2).

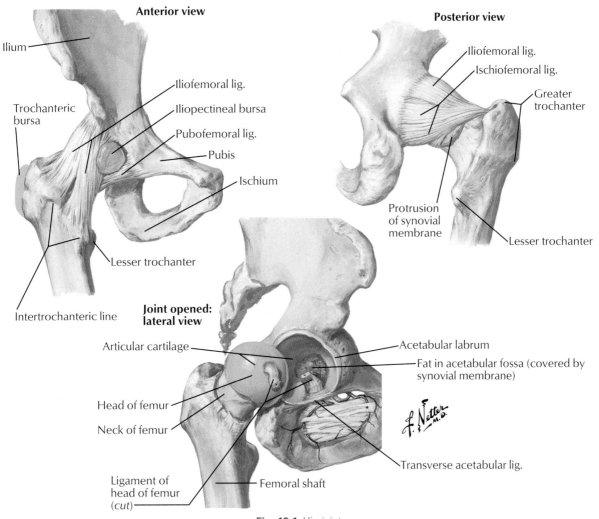

Anterior view

Ilium

Trochanteric bursa

Iliofemoral lig.

Iliopectineal bursa

Pubofemoral lig.

Pubis

Ischium

Lesser trochanter

Intertrochanteric line

Posterior view

Iliofemoral lig.

Ischiofemoral lig.

Greater trochanter

Protrusion of synovial membrane

Lesser trochanter

Joint opened: lateral view

Articular cartilage

Head of femur

Neck of femur

Ligament of head of femur (*cut*)

Acetabular labrum

Fat in acetabular fossa (covered by synovial membrane)

Transverse acetabular lig.

Femoral shaft

Fig. 13.1 Hip joint.

PRACTICE WHAT YOU PREACH 13.1
Wherefore Art Thou, Hip?

In exercise class, students may hear the instructor say, "Place your feet hip distance apart." The students will then assume a variety of positions because they often confuse the location of their hip joints (found medially) with their greater trochanters (found laterally). Find your actual hip-distance stance by first locating your hip joints near the groins and then placing your feet directly below.

PRACTICE WHAT YOU PREACH 13.2
Hip Hip, Hooray!

Which hip is your favorite? When standing for a prolonged period of time, we tend to lean to one side and bear much of our weight on that hip. This can lead to aches, pains, and muscular imbalances. So the next time you find yourself favoring one hip, adjust your stance to bear weight on both hips equally.

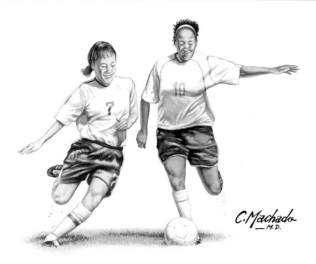

Fig. 13.2 "Wind-up" mechanism.

MOVEMENT

The multiaxial hip joint takes the thigh through an impressive array of movements: flexion, extension, abduction, adduction, and external and internal rotation (Fig. 13.3). Circumduction is also possible, a movement that uses all of the primary actions of the hip; it is seen when a dancer performs a fan kick. The hip can perform each of its main movements in different ways:

- **Femoral-on-pelvic movement**: As its name implies, in this mechanism, the femur moves within a relatively stationary pelvis. The movement is often employed for locomotion, as when the femur flexes and extends during walking.
- **Pelvic-on-femoral movement**: In this type of movement, the pelvis moves around a relatively stationary femur. It can happen in two ways:
  - **Long arc:** When the pelvis moves around the femur, the lumbar spine follows in the *same* direction, enabling a long arc of motion. This arc allows an increased range of motion of the trunk, enabling us, for example, to flex at the hip *and* bring the trunk closer to the ground to lift an object from the floor.
  - **Short arc:** When the pelvis moves around the femur, the lumbar spine moves in the *opposite* direction, creating a short arc of motion. This arc allows the lower extremities to move while the trunk remains stable. You employ this mechanism when you sit in a chair and stretch your back: your pelvis tilts anteriorly, while your lower back extends to keep your torso upright.

FLEXION

Remember your high school marching band? The band leader would parade across the football field, flexing his hips and raising his knees high. Hip flexion brings the anterior aspects of the thigh and pelvis closer together. This movement occurs in a couple of ways:

With femoral-on-pelvic flexion (illustrated in the marching band example), the femoral head rotates posteriorly, moving the femur anteriorly along the sagittal plane, while the pelvis stays stationary. Try **Moving AnatoME** with **Yoga Tree Pose (Vriksasana)** (see Video 13.1), and notice how, to enter into the pose, you engage your hip flexor muscles to flex your thigh as your torso remains stationary.

In comparison, pelvic-on-femoral movement occurs when your pelvis rotates anteriorly around the fixed femoral heads, simultaneously engaging the lower back extensor muscles to optimize alignment of the spine. Try **Moving AnatoME** with **Pilates Pelvic Tilts** (see Video 13.2) and work to keep your thighs stationary as your pelvis moves anteriorly and posteriorly to flex and extend your hips, respectively. Place one hand under your lower back and notice that, with an anterior pelvic tilt, the lumbar spine extends as your hips flex.

Approximate Range of Motion

80 degrees

Muscles and Innervation

See Fig. 13.4.

Muscle	Nerve
Psoas major	L1-L4
Iliacus	Femoral n. (L1-L4)
Rectus femoris	Femoral n. (L2-L4)
Sartorius	Femoral n. (L2, L3)
Tensor fasciae latae	Superior gluteal n. (L4, L5)
Pectineus	Femoral n. and obturator n. (L2-L4)
Adductor magnus (anterior part)	Obturator n. (L2-L4)
Adductor longus	Obturator n. (L2-L4)
Adductor brevis	Obturator n. (L2-L4)
Gracilis	Obturator n. (L2, L3)
Gluteus minimus (anterior fibers)	Superior gluteal n. (L5, S1)

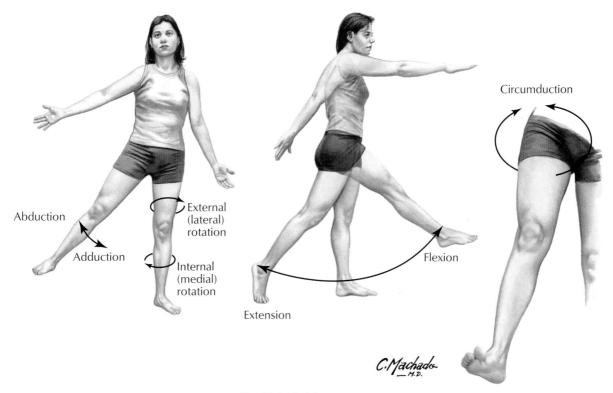

Circumduction

Abduction

External (lateral) rotation

Adduction

Internal (medial) rotation

Flexion

Extension

C. Machado _M.D.

Fig. 13.3 Hip joint movement.

Moving AnatoME Exercises

Hip Flexion (Femoral-on-Pelvic): Yoga Tree Pose (Vriksasana)

See Fig. 13.5 and Video 13.1.

- Starting position: Standing with your feet hip distance apart, in their natural parallel position. Weight is centered between both feet. Arms relax by your sides.
- Engage your core and shift your weight onto your right foot.
- Inhale and flex your left knee to lift your left foot. Then, abduct the thigh and externally rotate it to place the sole of your left foot on the inside of your right thigh (using your hands if necessary); your left toes should be pointing down toward the ground (modify by placing your foot on your calf or ankle and/or holding onto a nearby surface).
- Press your hands together in a prayer position (see Video 11.3) in front of your chest. When balanced, raise your arms overhead so they are parallel, with palms facing each other.

- For stability, press the sole of your left foot into your standing thigh and your thigh into your foot.
- Find a focus directly in front of you and maintain the position for five breaths.
- If elevated, return your palms to prayer position and lower your left foot to the ground.
- Repeat on the other side.
- Ending position: Relax your arms by your sides and return to a neutral stance.

Hip Flexion (Pelvic-on-Femoral): Pilates Pelvic Tilts

See Fig. 13.6, Video 13.2, and Clinical Focus 13.1.

- Starting position: Lying supine, with your legs hip distance apart, knees flexed, and feet flat on the floor. Arms are elongated by your sides with palms facing down. Your pelvis is in a neutral position, with the anterior superior iliac spines and pubic bone in the same plane, parallel to the floor; in this pelvic position, your lumbar spine maintains its natural lordotic curve (you can take one hand and place it underneath your lumbar spine to feel the space created by that curve).

CLINICAL FOCUS 13.1 Hip Replacement Surgery

Hip replacement surgery (hip arthroplasty) is performed hundreds of thousands of times a year. It is indicated for individuals with pain refractory to conservative treatment (eg, medication, physical therapy, corticosteroid injections). Common causes of such debilitating pain may include arthritis and hip fractures. Although movement is important for healing and to maintain mobility, certain joint positions, such as flexion of more than 90 degrees, can be contraindicated following surgery because they may lead to dislocation of the hip replacement depending on the type of incision and prosthetic used. Therefore, patients may need to modify their range of motion during exercise. In movements such as a runner's lunge or **Yoga Warrior II Pose** (see Video 13.8), for example, a postsurgical patient may need to decrease the degree of her lunge.

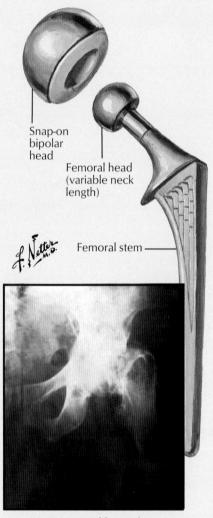

Snap-on bipolar head

Femoral head (variable neck length)

Femoral stem

Fracture of femoral neck with articular cartilage preserved

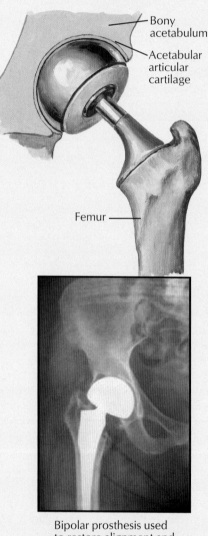

Bony acetabulum

Acetabular articular cartilage

Femur

Bipolar prosthesis used to restore alignment and function

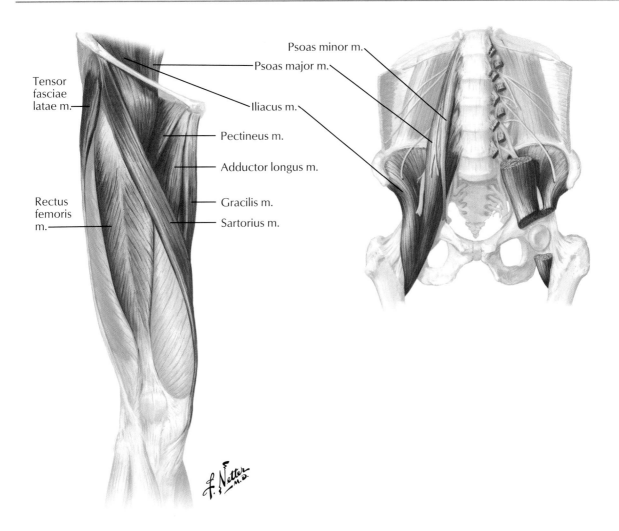

Tensor fasciae latae m.

Rectus femoris m.

Psoas minor m.
Psoas major m.
Iliacus m.
Pectineus m.
Adductor longus m.
Gracilis m.
Sartorius m.

Fig. 13.4 Muscles that flex the hip. (*Muscle not shown:* adductor magnus [anterior part].)

- Inhale to prepare.
- Exhale and engage your abdominals to flex your lumbar spine, extend your hips, and tilt your pelvis posteriorly so that your pubic bone is more superior than your anterior superior iliac spines.
- Inhale and begin to slowly extend the lumbar spine, restoring its lordotic curve, and flexing your hips to return your pelvis to a neutral position.
- Repeat six to eight times, moving back and forth from a neutral to posteriorly tilted pelvis.
- Ending position: Lying supine with your back and pelvis in their neutral position.

EXTENSION

Our society spends a lot of time sitting (see Hamstring Strain, Clinical Focus 13.2). If you are currently in a seated position, stand up to stretch your legs. To do this, you extend not only your knee but also your hip. In hip extension, the distance between the posterior aspects of the femur and pelvis decreases. Similar to flexion, extension occurs via two main mechanisms. The aforementioned example of standing up from a seated position employs femoral-on-pelvic extension, with the femoral head rolling anteriorly to move its shaft posteriorly within

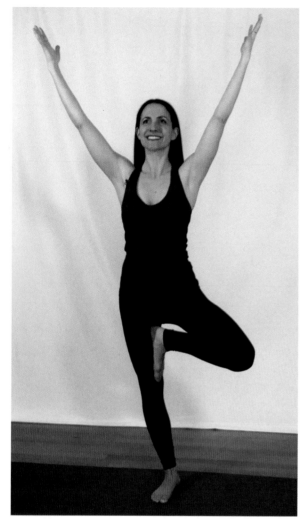

Fig. 13.5 Hip flexion (femoral-on-pelvic): **Yoga Tree Pose (Vriksasana)** (see Video 13.1).

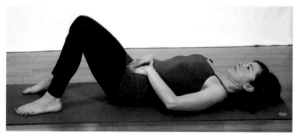

Fig. 13.6 Hip flexion (pelvic-on-femoral): **Pilates Pelvic Tilts** (see Video 13.2).

the sagittal plane, while the pelvis remains stationary. Try **Moving AnatoME** with **Pilates Swimming** (see Video 13.3). As you enter into the exercise, try to isolate the engagement of your hamstring and gluteal muscles and refrain from clenching your lumbar extensors, a common mistake.

In contrast, pelvic-on-femoral extension is just the opposite motion; it occurs when your pelvis rotates posteriorly around fixed femoral heads. Try **Moving AnatoME** with **Pilates Pelvic Tilts** (see Video 13.2), and work to keep your thighs stationary as your pelvis moves anteriorly and posteriorly to flex and extend your hips, respectively. Place one hand under your lower back, and notice that, with a posterior pelvic tilt, the lumbar spine flexes as your hips extend.

Approximate Range of Motion

20 degrees

Muscles and Innervation

See Fig. 13.7.

Muscle	Nerve
Gluteus maximus	Inferior gluteal n. (L5-S2)
Biceps femoris (long head)	Tibial division of sciatic n. (L5- S2)
Semitendinosus	Tibial division of sciatic n. (L5-S2)
Semimembranosus	Tibial division of sciatic n. (L5- S2)
Adductor magnus (posterior head)	Tibial division of sciatic n. (L4)
Gluteus medius (posterior fibers)	Superior gluteal n. (L5, S1)

Moving AnatoME Exercises
Hip Extension (Femoral-on-Pelvic):
Pilates Swimming

See Fig. 13.8 and Video 13.3.

• Starting position: Lying prone on the floor. Your shoulders are flexed and forearms pronated, with palms facing down and fingertips reaching in front of you. Your legs are hip distance apart, thighs externally rotated, knees extended and ankles plantarflexed; the dorsal surfaces of your feet lengthen along the floor. Your spine and pelvis are neutral, with your core engaged.

• Inhale to prepare.

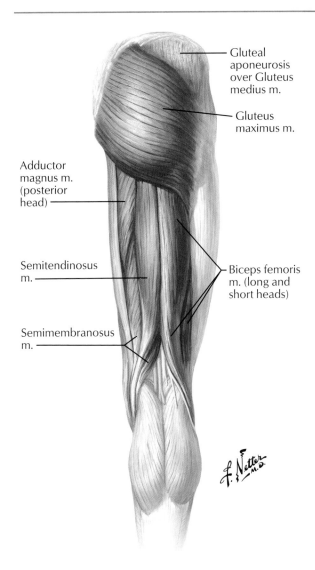

Gluteal aponeurosis over Gluteus medius m.

Gluteus maximus m.

Adductor magnus m. (posterior head)

Semitendinosus m.

Biceps femoris m. (long and short heads)

Semimembranosus m.

Fig. 13.7 Muscles that extend the hip.

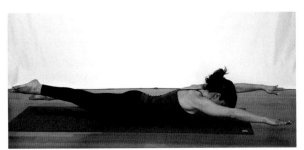

Fig. 13.8 Hip extension (femoral-on-pelvic): **Pilates Swimming** (see Video 13.3).

- Exhale and slowly extend your thighs to lift them off the ground without moving your pelvis. Simultaneously extend the thorax to lift the torso off the ground. Keep your cervical spine in line with your thoracic spine and your gaze toward your mat.
- As you maintain this position and avoid rotation of the vertebral column or pelvis, "swim" opposite arms and legs by flexing and extending the contralateral shoulder and hip joints with small and controlled motions, inhaling for five counts and exhaling for five counts.
- Repeat for five total cycles of inhaling and exhaling.
- Ending position: Slowly lower your arms, legs, and torso to the floor.

Hip Extension (Pelvic-on-Femoral): Pilates Pelvic Tilts

See Fig. 13.9, Video 13.2, and Clinical Focus 13.2; see **Hip Flexion (Pelvic-on-Femoral)** for exercise steps.

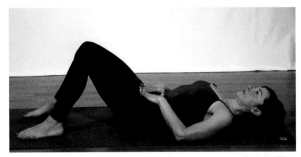

Fig. 13.9 Hip extension (pelvic-on-femoral): **Pilates Pelvic Tilts** (see Video 13.2).

ABDUCTION

Stand with your feet together. Now jump your feet sideways, apart from each other, as if you were doing a jumping-jack. You just abducted both of your thighs at your hip joints, reducing the distance between the lateral aspect of each thigh and the iliac crest.

This type of abduction is called femoral-on-pelvic abduction. The head of the femur glides inferiorly, allowing the femoral shaft to rise laterally along the frontal plane, while the pelvis remains relatively stationary. Try **Moving AnatoME** with **Pilates Side Leg Series (Abduction)** (see Video 13.4). Place your hand on your gluteal region during this exercise, and feel your abductors engage.

CLINICAL FOCUS 13.2
Hamstring Strain

Hamstring strain refers to a tear of one or more of the posterior muscles of the thigh (biceps femoris, semi-tendinosus, semimembranosus). Risk factors such as muscle tightness, weakness, and imbalance predispose an individual to this injury. In modern society, a common cause of muscular imbalance is prolonged sitting. Whether at work, at home, or in the car, sitting for long periods of time can tighten the hip flexor muscles and weaken the extensor muscles, especially the gluteus maximus muscle. When the gluteus maximus elongates and weakens, the hamstring muscles compensate, even though they are intended to work as synergists and not prime movers. Indeed, overloading the hamstrings is a common mechanism of muscle strain, with ripple effects on gait, posture, and overall movement patterns. Regular, gentle hip strengthening exercises such as **Pilates Swimming** (see Video 13.3) can help keep the hip extensor muscles strong, restore muscular balance to the region, and prevent injury.

A second way to abduct the thigh involves a stationary femur and a pelvis rotating laterally around it in the frontal plane. You employ pelvic-on-femoral abduction every day when walking; your abductors support your standing leg, and your torso upright upon it, as the other leg swings off the ground. Without this abduction, the pelvis and trunk would drop toward the side of the swinging limb. Try **Moving AnatoME** with **Yoga Triangle Pose (Trikonasana)** (see Video 13.5). Tune into the action of your pelvis rotating around a stationary femur, as your torso leans toward the floor. Remember to anchor your back foot on the ground as your weight shifts.

Approximate Range of Motion
40 degrees

Muscles and Innervation
See Fig. 13.10.

Muscle	Nerve
Gluteus medius	Superior gluteal n. (L5, S1)
Gluteus minimus	Superior gluteal n. (L5, S1)
Tensor fasciae latae	Superior gluteal n. (L4, L5)
Sartorius	Femoral n. (L2, L3)
Piriformis	S1, S2 (ventral rami)

Moving AnatoME Exercises
Hip Abduction (Femoral-on-Pelvic): Pilates Side Leg Series (Abduction)
See Fig. 13.11 and Video 13.4.

- Starting position: Lying on your left side in one long line, with shoulders, hips, knees, and ankles aligned from head to toe. Place your top hand on the floor in front of your torso for support; your bottom shoulder is flexed, and, depending on comfort, your bottom elbow is either extended with your head resting on your arm or is flexed with your head resting on your hand. Engage your core to prevent your torso from rocking back and forth (imagine that you are between two panes of glass).
- Inhale, plantarflex the top foot, and abduct the top hip until the top leg is just a little higher than hip height.
- Exhale and dorsiflex the top foot, reaching through your heel as you adduct the top hip and return the leg to its starting position.
- Repeat six to eight times, and then perform on the other side.
- Ending position: Lying comfortably on your side.

Hip Abduction (Pelvic-on-Femoral): Yoga Triangle Pose (Trikonasana)
See Fig. 13.12, Video 13.5, and Clinical Focus 13.3.

- Starting position: Standing with your feet hip distance apart, in their natural parallel position. Weight is centered between both feet. Arms relax by your sides.
- Abduct your arms to 90 degrees, and step your feet apart so that your ankles align under your wrists. Depress your scapulae, maintain a neutral wrist, and extend the fingers.
- Turn your left foot slightly inward (15 to 45 degrees) and your right foot 90 degrees outward. Align your left and right heels.
- Exhale, ground your left foot on the floor, and abduct at the right hip as you laterally flex your torso, aiming to bring the right lateral aspect of your torso parallel to the ground with shoulders stacked in one plane (avoid rotating, flexing, or hyperextending your spine). Engage your core, initiating slight lumbar flexion to draw the pelvis into a slight posterior tilt.
- Place your right hand on the floor outside of your right foot; if this is not possible, place it on your ankle or shin. Lift your left arm toward the ceiling, in line

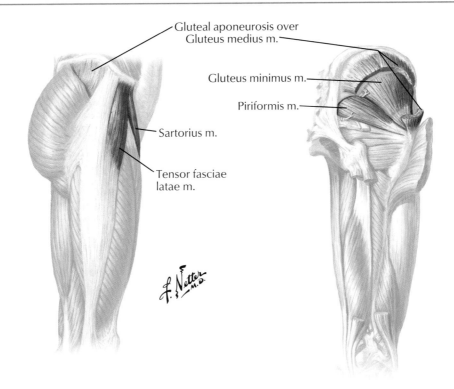

Gluteal aponeurosis over
Gluteus medius m.

Gluteus minimus m.

Piriformis m.

Sartorius m.

Tensor fasciae
latae m.

Fig. 13.10 Muscles that abduct the hip.

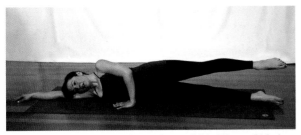

Fig. 13.11 Hip abduction (femoral-on-pelvic): **Pilates Side Leg Series (Abduction)** (see Video 13.4).

with your shoulders. If possible, rotate your head to gaze toward the left hand.
- Maintain this position for five easy breaths.
- Ground the left foot and inhale, returning your torso to neutral as you adduct the right hip.
- Reverse sides.
- Ending position: From the final neutral position, exhale, lower your arms, and step your feet back into a hip-distance stance.

ADDUCTION

When you sit down, do you cross your legs? This posture involves adduction of your thighs, in which the medial aspect of the femur moves toward or past the midline of the body. It can happen in one of two ways:

In the aforementioned example, adduction occurs by a femoral-on-pelvic mechanism; as the femoral head glides superiorly, the shaft of the femur moves medially along the frontal plane while the pelvis remains relatively stationary. Try **Moving AnatoME** with **Pilates Side Leg Series (Adduction)** (see Video 13.6), and feel the muscles in your inner thighs work against gravity to bring your thighs together.

Additionally, pelvic-on-femoral adduction occurs when your femur remains stationary and your pelvis rotates medially around it in the frontal plane. To isolate this movement, stand on your right leg and drop the left side of your pelvis toward the floor, decreasing the length of your right waist and bringing your right hip into adduction. Try **Moving AnatoME** with **Yoga Triangle Pose (Trikonasana)** (see Video 13.5). As you exit the pose and return your torso to an upright position, you are adducting the front hip.

CLINICAL FOCUS 13.3   **Trochanteric Bursitis**

A bursa is a small fluid-filled sac that reduces friction between two surfaces. The trochanteric bursa, for example, cushions the tendons of gluteal muscles from the bony prominence of the greater trochanter. Because bursae are found in high friction areas, they are easily overworked and can become inflamed, eventually leading to bursitis. Stressors like trauma, overuse, and postural imbalances can cause bursitis. Because many laypeople refer to the outer portion of the thigh as the hip, a patient with bursitis may talk about hip pain when consulting a physician. Although trochanteric bursitis is often thought of as a cause of "hip"

pain, the trochanter is not actually part of the hip joint. Therefore, bursitis in the region does not cause true joint pain. In addition to "hip pain," patients may also describe difficulty in sleeping on the affected side, and also may refer to pain during jogging, stair climbing, or cross-legged sitting, activities that further aggravate the bursa. Because several of the gluteal muscles are thigh abductors, stretching this muscle group can help relieve compression and irritation. Strengthening exercises such as the **Pilates Side Leg Series** (see Video 13.4) can help stabilize the region and prevent further muscular imbalances.

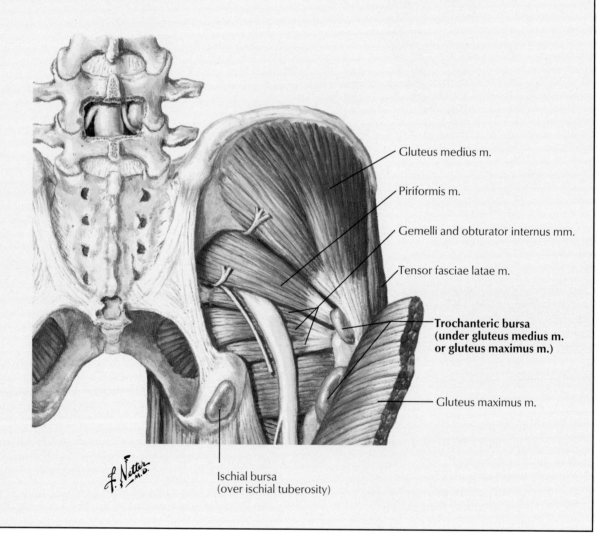

Gluteus medius m.

Piriformis m.

Gemelli and obturator internus mm.

Tensor fasciae latae m.

Trochanteric bursa (under gluteus medius m. or gluteus maximus m.)

Gluteus maximus m.

Ischial bursa (over ischial tuberosity)

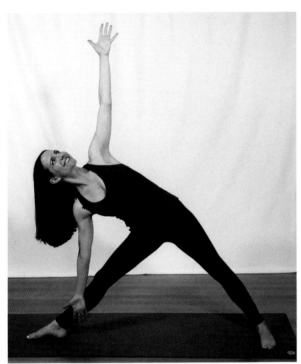

Fig. 13.12 Hip abduction (pelvic-on-femoral): **Yoga Triangle Pose (Trikonasana)** (see Video 13.5).

Approximate Range of Motion

25 degrees

Muscles and Innervation

See Fig. 13.13.

Muscle	Nerve
Adductor magnus	Anterior head: obturator n. (L2-L4)
	Posterior head: tibial part of sciatic n. (L4)
Adductor longus	Obturator n. (L2-L4)
Adductor brevis	Obturator n. (L2-L4)
Gracilis	Obturator n. (L2, L3)
Pectineus	Femoral n. and obturator n. (L2-L4)
Biceps femoris (long head)	Tibial division of sciatic n. (L5-S2)
Quadratus femoris	Nerve to quadratus femoris (L5, S1)
Gluteus maximus (lower fibers)	Inferior gluteal n. (L5-S2)

Moving AnatoME Exercises

Hip Adduction (Femoral-on-Pelvic): Pilates Side Leg Series (Adduction)

See Fig. 13.14 and Video 13.6.

- Starting position: Lying on your left side in one long line, with shoulders, hips, knees, and ankles aligned from head to toe. Place your top hand on the floor in front of your torso for support; your bottom shoulder is flexed and, depending on comfort, your bottom elbow is either extended with your head resting on your arm or is flexed with your head resting on your hand. Engage your core to prevent your torso from rocking back and forth (imagine that you are between two panes of glass).
- Inhale to plantarflex the top foot and abduct the top thigh to your hip height.
- Exhale, engage your core, and adduct the bottom hip, bringing the bottom thigh up to meet the top thigh. Continue exhaling as you lower both legs back to the floor simultaneously.
- Repeat six to eight times, and then perform on the other side.
- Ending position: Lying comfortably on your side.

Hip Adduction (Pelvic-on-Femoral): Yoga Triangle Pose (Trikonasana)

See Fig. 13.12 and Video 13.5; see **Hip Abduction (Pelvic-on-Femoral)** for exercise text.

EXTERNAL ROTATION

Stand in anatomical position, with your feet parallel to each other. Now place your feet into a dancer's first position, by sliding your heels together so that your toes point diagonally outward. To arrive in first position, you externally rotated your thighs, turning the anterior aspect of the thigh away from the midline.

External rotation of the hip occurs in two main ways. Typically, it occurs with femoral-on-pelvic rotation, as seen when you assume first position. The movement occurs as the femur rolls laterally about a longitudinal axis while the pelvis remains stable. Try **Moving AnatoME** with the **Pilates Clamshell** (see Video 13.7) exercise. Make sure that your seat is stable before you externally rotate your thighs. Only rotate them as far as you are able to retain an erect spine.

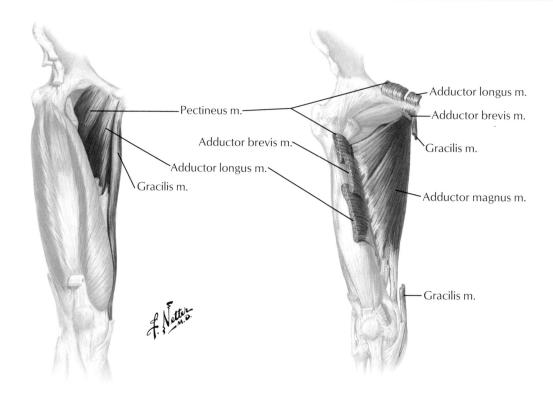

Fig. 13.13 Muscles that adduct the hip. (*Muscle not shown:* quadratus femoris.)

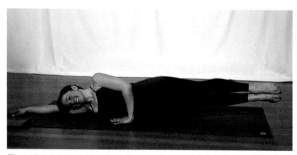

Fig. 13.14 Hip adduction (femoral-on-pelvic): **Pilates Side Leg Series (Adduction)** (see Video 13.6).

In pelvic-on-femoral rotation, the femur remains stable while the pelvis rotates medially around it. We employ this motion commonly when pivoting to quickly change directions. See for yourself: Plant your right foot firmly on the ground and then cut to the left; notice that by rotating your pelvis to the left about your fixed right femur, you externally rotated your right hip.

Try **Moving AnatoME** with **Warrior II Pose** (see Video 13.8). Note that the front hip is externally rotated, via femoral-on-pelvic rotation. Additionally, a small amount of pelvic-on-femoral external rotation in the back hip may be required to bring both hips into alignment.

Approximate Range of Motion

45 degrees

Muscles and Innervation

See Fig. 13.15.

Muscle	Nerve
Gluteus maximus	Inferior gluteal n. (L5-S2)
Sartorius	Femoral n. (L2, L3)
Piriformis (see Clinical Focus 13.4)	S1, S2 (ventral rami)
Gemellus superior	Nerve to obturator internus (L5, S1)

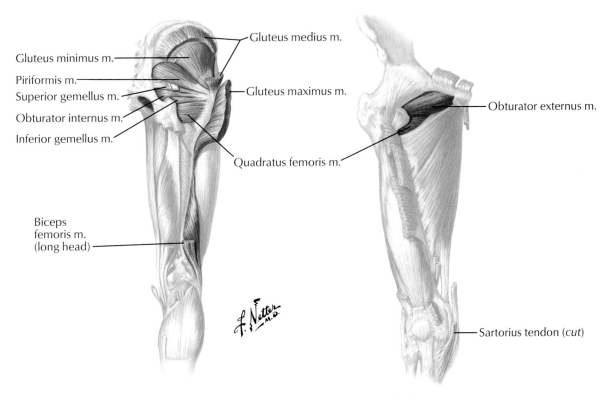

Gluteus medius m.

Gluteus minimus m.

Piriformis m.

Superior gemellus m.

Obturator internus m.

Inferior gemellus m.

Gluteus maximus m.

Obturator externus m.

Quadratus femoris m.

Biceps
femoris m.
(long head)

Sartorius tendon (*cut*)

Fig. 13.15 Muscles that externally rotate the hip.

Muscle	Nerve
Gemellus inferior	Nerve to quadratus femoris (L5, S1)
Obturator internus	Nerve to obturator internus (L5, S1)
Obturator externus	Obturator n. (L3, L4)
Quadratus femoris	Nerve to quadratus femoris (L5, S1)
Gluteus medius (posterior fibers)	Superior gluteal n. (L5, S1)
Gluteus minimus (posterior fibers)	Superior gluteal n. (L5, S1)
Biceps femoris, long head	Tibial division of sciatic n. (L5-S2)

Moving AnatoME Exercises
Hip External Rotation (Femoral-on-Pelvic): Pilates Clamshell
▶ See Fig. 13.16 and Video 13.7.
- Starting position: Lying on your left side with your knees flexed, ankles stacked, and heels in line with hips and shoulders. Place your top hand on the floor in front of your torso for support; your bottom shoulder is flexed and, depending on comfort, your bottom elbow is either extended with your head resting on your arm or is flexed with your head resting on your hand. Engage your core to prevent your torso from rocking back and forth.
- Inhale to prepare.
- Exhale, draw your navel in, and externally rotate the top hip to open the top thigh like a clamshell. Keep the medial aspects of the feet connected, and reach the top knee toward the ceiling only as far as you can maintain a neutral pelvis to isolate femoral-on-pelvic rotation.
- Inhale and internally rotate the top thigh, returning the top knee to its starting position. Control the movement by resisting gravity as you slowly lower the thigh.
- Ending position: Lying comfortably on your side.

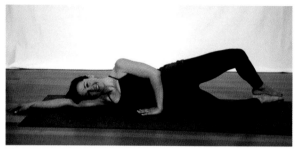

Fig. 13.16 Hip external rotation (femoral-on-pelvic): **Pilates Clamshell** (see Video 13.7).

Hip External Rotation (Pelvic-on-Femoral): Yoga Warrior II Pose (Virabhadrasana II)

▶ See Fig. 13.17, Video 13.8, and Clinical Focus 13.4.

- Starting position: Standing with your feet hip distance apart, in their natural parallel position. Weight is centered between both feet. Arms relax by your sides.
- Abduct your arms to 90 degrees, and step your feet apart so that your ankles align under your wrists. Keep your shoulders down, wrists neutral, and fingers elongated.
- Turn your left foot slightly inward (15 to 45 degrees) and your right foot 90 degrees outward. Align your left and right heels.
- Flex your right knee to 90 degrees, so that your thigh comes parallel to the floor. Position your knee directly over your ankle and aligned with your second toe. Ground all four corners of each foot and lift your arches.

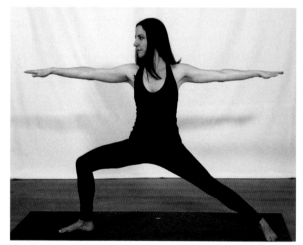

Fig. 13.17 Hip external rotation (pelvic-on-femoral): **Yoga Warrior II Pose (Virabhadrasana II)** (see Video 13.8).

CLINICAL FOCUS 13.4
Piriformis Syndrome

The piriformis is a small muscle located deep in the gluteal region that externally rotates the hip. Under (and sometimes through) this muscle courses the sciatic nerve as it travels down the posterior thigh and leg. If the piriformis tightens, spasms, or hypertrophies, or if the surrounding soft tissue becomes inflamed, compression of the sciatic nerve can occur, causing sciatic-like symptoms. For example, patients may report buttock pain that can also radiate to the posterior thigh. Runners who overuse the muscle are more likely to experience the syndrome, as are women whose posture becomes hyperlordotic during pregnancy. Exercises such as **Yoga Half Lord of the Fishes Pose** (Video 16.2) can help keep the piriformis and surrounding musculature properly stretched and less likely to cause compression.

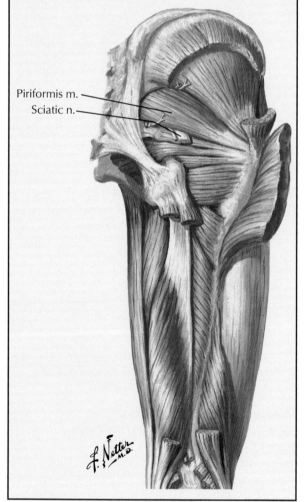

Piriformis m.
Sciatic n.

- Rotate your head to gaze over your right fingertips. Your torso should remain upright; it should not be leaning forward.
- Stay in this position for five slow and deliberate breaths.
- Extend your right knee, reverse directions, and repeat to the left side.
- Ending position: Rotate your head to neutral, relax your arms, straighten both knees, and step your feet into a hip distance stance.

INTERNAL ROTATION

From a dancer's first position (see **External Rotation** earlier in chapter), slide your toes in toward the midline, bringing your feet into a parallel position. To do this, you internally rotated your hips, turning the anterior aspect of the thighs toward the midline. Internal rotation is very similar to external rotation, employing the same mechanisms in reverse directions. By assuming parallel position, you demonstrated femoral-on-pelvic rotation, which occurs when the femur rolls medially about a longitudinal axis while the pelvis remains fixed. Try **Moving AnatoME** with **Pilates Clamshell** (see Video 13.7). Lower your thigh with control, creating your own resistance to feel the engagement of your internal rotators.

A subtler form of internal rotation, pelvic-on-femoral, is seen when walking. During the stance phase, the femur is fixed and the pelvis rotates laterally around it. This movement is only a few degrees, but it happens regularly during locomotion to decouple pelvic and trunk motion, so the shoulders can remain square while the lower limbs ambulate. Try **Moving AnatoME** with **Warrior I Pose** (see Video 13.9). Notice the fine-tuning internal rotation that occurs in your front hip as you square your pelvis to the front edge of your mat (Box 13.1).

Approximate Range of Motion
35 degrees

Muscles and Innervation
See Fig. 13.18.

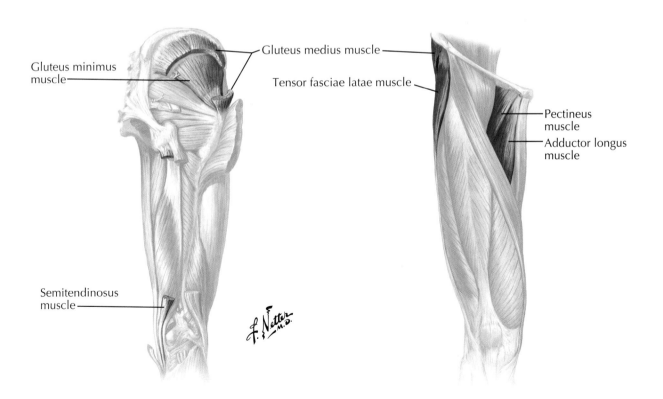

Fig. 13.18 Muscles that internally rotate the hip. (*Muscle not shown:* adductor brevis.)

Muscle	Nerve
Gluteus medius (anterior fibers)	Superior gluteal n. (L5, S1)
Gluteus minimus (anterior fibers)	Superior gluteal n. (L5, S1)
Tensor fasciae latae	Superior gluteal n. (L4, L5)
Pectineus	Femoral n. and obturator n. (L2-L4)
Adductor longus	Obturator n. (L2, L3, L4)
Adductor brevis	Obturator n. (L2, L3, L4)
Semitendinosus	Tibial division of sciatic n. (L5-S2)
Semimembranosus	Tibial division of sciatic n. (L5-S2)

BOX 13.1   The Inside Scoop on Internal Rotation

Although you may not go to the gym or a fitness class to intentionally strengthen your internal rotator muscles, you frequently employ internal rotation to maintain proper alignment during exercise. Often times, this is required to counteract the pull of external rotator muscles, which tend to be stronger and better developed. Often times, external rotators are stronger than internal rotators and, due to this muscular imbalance, you may need to engage your internal rotators to restore alignment during an exercise. For instance, the **Yoga Seated Forward Fold** (see Video 15.1) does not necessitate internal rotation of the thighs; depending on your muscular imbalances, however, to keep your thighs parallel to each other you might need to engage your internal rotator muscles.

Moving AnatoME Exercises
Hip Internal Rotation (Femoral-on-Pelvic): Pilates Clamshell

See Fig. 13.19 and Video 13.7; see **Hip External Rotation (Femoral-on-Pelvic)** for exercise steps.

Hip Internal Rotation (Pelvic-on-Femoral): Yoga Warrior I Pose (Virabhadrasana I)

See Fig. 13.20 and Video 13.9.
- Starting position: Standing with your feet hip distance apart, in their natural parallel position. Weight is centered between both feet. Arms relax by your sides.
- Inhale and step your feet 3 to 4 feet apart so that your ankles align under your wrists. Abduct your arms to 180 degrees, and externally rotate your shoulders so that your palms face each other. Keep your scapulae depressed, wrists neutral, and fingers extended.

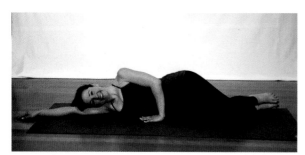

Fig. 13.19 Hip internal rotation (femoral-on-pelvic): **Pilates Clamshell** (see Video 13.7).

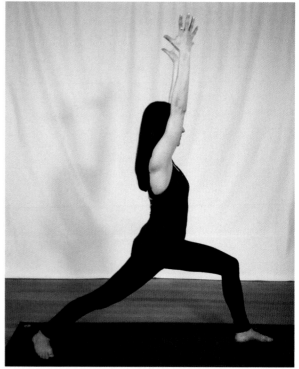

Fig. 13.20 Hip internal rotation (pelvic-on-femoral): **Yoga Warrior I Pose (Virabhadrasana I)** (see Video 13.9).

- Turn your left foot inward (45 to 60 degrees) and your right foot 90 degrees outward. Align your left and right heels.
- Exhale and flex your right knee so that the thigh comes parallel to the floor. Position your knee directly over your ankle and aligned with your second toe. Ground all four corners of your front foot and lift the arch. Rotate your torso to the right, internally rotating the left hip to square your pelvis as much as possible toward the front edge of your mat; ground the lateral aspect of the left foot and lift its arch.
- Inhale and extend your spine. Keep your head in a neutral position, or extend it slightly to elevate your gaze.
- Stay in this position for five slow, deep breaths.
- Extend your right knee, reverse directions, and repeat to the left side.
- Ending position: Inhale, straighten the left knee, and release your arms. Return your feet to a hip-distance stance.

14

Knee

OVERVIEW

- The knee is a modified hinge joint that connects the thigh and leg.
- Its articulations occur between the femur and patella (the patellofemoral joint) and the femur and tibia (the tibiofemoral joint).
- Movements include flexion, extension, and rotation.
- Movements occur in two ways: femoral-on-tibial and tibial-on-femoral.
- Example exercises:
  - Flexion (**Pilates Single Leg Kick,** Video 14.1; **Yoga Chair Pose,** Video 14.2)
  - Extension (**Pilates Single Leg Kick,** Video 14.1; **Yoga Chair Pose,** Video 14.2)

STRUCTURE AND FUNCTION

Sit down and place your hands on your knees. These smooth, simple surfaces (your patella bones, a.k.a. kneecaps) belie the sophisticated joints below them. Each synovial knee joint is a modified hinge that is composed of three bones, the patella, femur, and tibia (Fig. 14.1A). Together, these bones form two articulations: The patella rests within the intercondylar groove of the femur to form the patellofemoral joint, and the condyles of the femur articulate with the smaller condyles of the tibia to form the tibiofemoral joint. Note that the fibula, although it is in close proximity to the tibia, is not part of the knee joint (it is a common misconception to think that it is). The fibula does play a role at the knee by serving as an attachment site for structures that cross the knee joint, such as the biceps femoris tendon and the lateral collateral ligament. By virtue of its position, it also helps maintain the tibia's alignment.

The tibia and fibula articulate at the proximal tibiofemoral joint. The connection between the tibia and fibula continues via an interosseous membrane that helps expand the surface area and transmit biomechanical forces; it terminates in the syndesmotic distal tibiofemoral articulation, which forms a portion of the ankle joint.

The knee's dual-joint composition balances stability and mobility as you stand, jog, jump, and climb stairs every day. Stability is an important consideration given that the synovial joint, even though it is the largest in the body, is a relatively small articulation compared with the large amount of stress it bears (compressive forces on the joint regularly reach two to three times your body's weight). To ensure maximal stability, the knee relies on soft tissue structures, such as the medial/lateral collateral and anterior/posterior cruciate ligaments, and large muscles, which heavily reinforce the joint capsule. The medial (C-shaped) and lateral (O-shaped) menisci, which are fibrocartilaginous shock absorbers that almost triple the joint's surface area, also stabilize the joint, as well as cushion it and reduce pressure on it. This support helps the tibiofemoral—and especially the tibia—transfer weight across the knee to the ankle. The patellofemoral joint additionally lightens the load by acting as a pulley system. The patella is the largest sesamoid bone in the body, sheathed in the tendon of the quadratus femoris muscle. It increases the lever arm of the quadriceps muscle, which decreases the amount of energy required to move the leg, thereby increasing the muscular strength on it (see Fig. 14.1B).

In terms of mobility, the knee mainly performs extension and flexion. It is not a simple hinge joint, however (if it were, only flexion and extension would be possible). It is a modified joint, permitting gliding and rotation, as well; these are subtle movements that occur when the

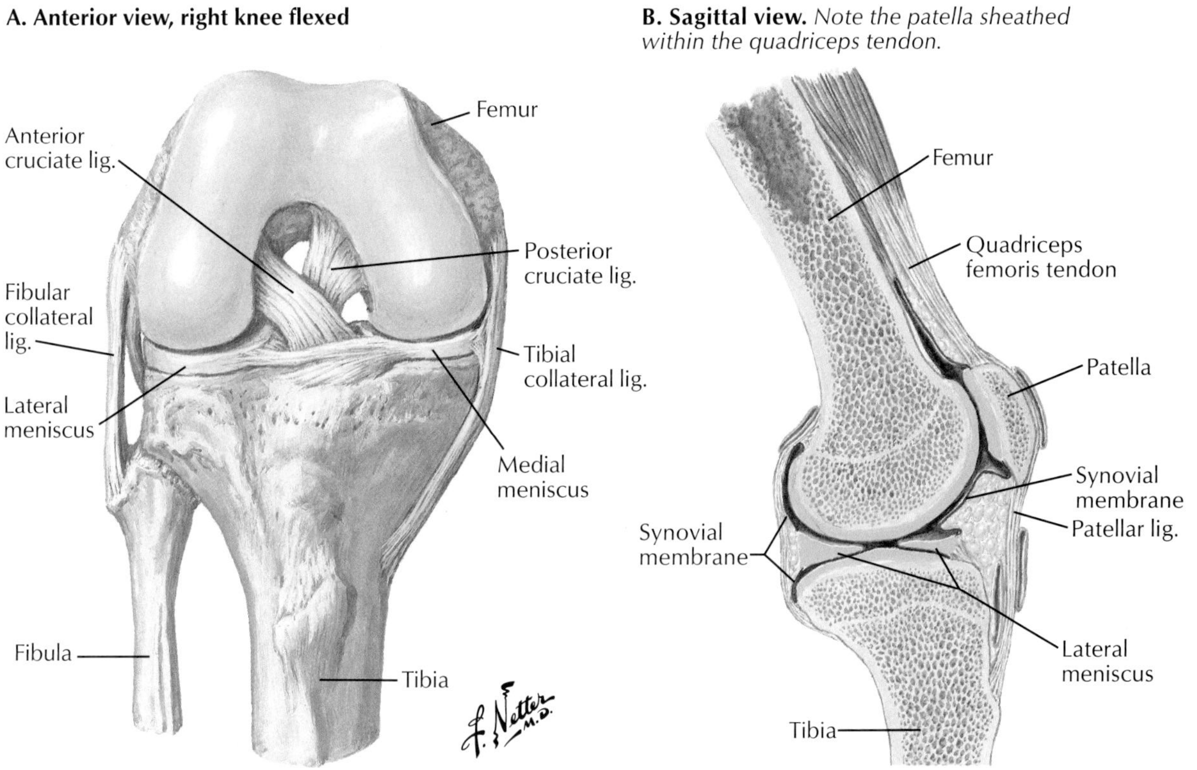

A. Anterior view, right knee flexed

B. Sagittal view. *Note the patella sheathed within the quadriceps tendon.*

Femur

Anterior cruciate lig.

Posterior cruciate lig.

Fibular collateral lig.

Tibial collateral lig.

Lateral meniscus

Medial meniscus

Fibula

Tibia

Femur

Quadriceps femoris tendon

Patella

Synovial membrane

Patellar lig.

Synovial membrane

Lateral meniscus

Tibia

Fig. 14.1. Knee joint.

knee is flexed (see Fig. 14.2). In addition to having its own movements, the knee is affected by the motions of the hip above and the ankle below; indeed, several muscles that move the knee also cross the hip or ankle (eg, the sartorius and gastrocnemius, respectively). It is easy to see, then, how misalignment in one joint can cause dysfunction of other joints in the biomechanical chain; for instance, hip injury or an ankle sprain can lead to knee pain.

MOVEMENT

Muscles found in both the thigh and the leg act on the knee to create flexion and extension, along with slight internal and external rotation when the knee is flexed (Fig. 14.2). Flexion and extension involve three synergistic mechanisms: rolling and sliding at the tibiofemoral joint, gliding at the patellofemoral joint, and natural rotation at the articular surfaces. Surrounding structures of the knee limit its movements, for example, tension of the collateral and cruciate ligaments limits the range of

extension; soft tissues on the posterior leg and thigh, as well as tension in the quadriceps muscle group, help determine the range of flexion.

Flexion and extension can occur in two different ways:
- **Femoral-on-tibial movement**: As its name implies, this closed-chain mechanism involves the femur moving on a relatively stationary tibia. It is employed, for instance, when one sits down on a chair, as the femur flexes upon a fixed tibia.
- **Tibial-on-femoral movement**: This open-chain movement involves the tibia moving around a relatively stationary femur, as occurs when one is running down the street or kicking a soccer ball.

FLEXION

If you're an average American, you may sit for 10 hours per day. To sit, you flex your knees, bringing your posterior leg and thigh closer together. Knee flexion occurs in two ways. During tibial-on-femoral flexion, the tibial condyles roll and slide posteriorly over stationary femoral condyles

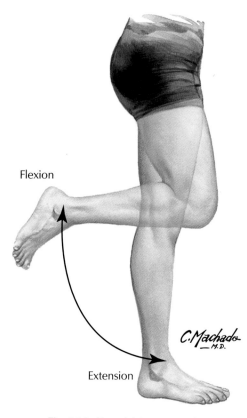

Flexion

Extension

C. Machado
—M.D.

Fig. 14.2. Knee joint movement.

moderate external rotation of the femur (in femoral-on-tibial flexion) or internal rotation of the tibia (in tibial-on-femoral flexion). The second type is a rotation that can occur independently between the tibia and femur when the knee is in partial flexion, allowing for external and internal rotation of the tibia on the horizontal plane. You may have seen this performed on a rotator disc at a Pilates studio, or on the soccer field when a player "cuts." Internal rotation is a more powerful movement than its external counterpart; indeed, many more muscles are responsible for internal rotation (ie, the semimembranosus, semitendinosus, gracilis, sartorius, and popliteus muscles) than external rotation (ie, the biceps femoris muscle).

Approximate Range of Motion

140 degrees

Muscles and Innervation

See Fig. 14.3.

Muscle	Nerve
Hamstrings	
Semimembranosus	Tibial branch of sciatic n. (L4-S2)
Semitendinosus	Tibial branch of sciatic n. (L4-S2)
Biceps femoris, long head and short head	Tibial branch of sciatic n. (L5-S3); fibular branch of sciatic n. (L5-S2)
Sartorius	Femoral n. (L2, S3)
Gracilis	Obturator n. (L2, S3)
Gastrocnemius	Tibial n. (S1, S2)
Plantaris	Tibial n. (S1, S2)
Popliteus	Tibial n. (L4-S1)

at the tibiofemoral joint while the patella concurrently glides distally at the patellofemoral joint; this moves the leg posteriorly along the sagittal plane. Try **Moving AnatoME** with **Pilates Single Leg Kick** (see Video 14.1). As you bend your knees, keep your thighs stationary to isolate movement of the tibia.

During femoral-on-tibial flexion, the femoral condyles roll posteriorly and slide anteriorly over stationary tibial condyles, as the patella glides distally. Try **Moving AnatoME** with **Yoga Chair Pose** (**Utkatasana**) (see Video 14.2). As you enter into the pose, keep your legs stationary. Shift weight into your heels and sit back as if you were sitting on a chair, bringing your knees into flexion by moving only your femurs.

Accompanying flexion are two types of rotation. The first type is an automatic rotation that occurs during active knee flexion to unlock an extended knee. Initiated by the popliteus muscle, this rotation can result in a

Moving AnatoME Exercises
Knee Flexion (Tibial-on-Femoral):
Pilates Single Leg Kick

See Fig. 14.4 and Video 14.1.
- Starting position: Lying prone, with your lumbar and thoracic spines extended and cervical spine neutral; elbows are flexed and placed directly under your shoulders to support your torso. Your forearms are parallel and facing the midline; fingers are flexed. Engage your core to protect your lower back. Isometrically press into the floor with your forearms and flexed hands to stabilize the upper body.

Superficial dissection   Deep dissection

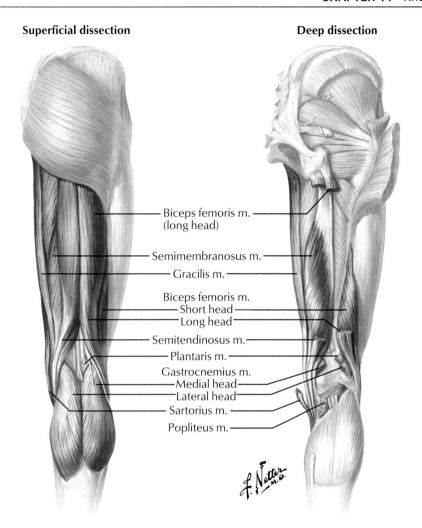

Biceps femoris m.
(long head)

Semimembranosus m.

Gracilis m.

Biceps femoris m.
Short head
Long head
Semitendinosus m.
Plantaris m.
Gastrocnemius m.
Medial head
Lateral head
Sartorius m.
Popliteus m.

Fig. 14.3. Muscles that flex the knee.

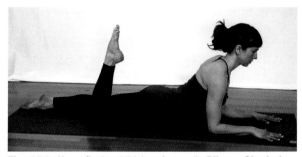

Fig. 14.4. Knee flexion (tibial-on-femoral): **Pilates Single Leg Kick** (see Video 14.1).

- Inhale to prepare.
- Exhale, flex the right knee, and pulse twice, plantarflexing the ankle on the first pulse and dorsiflexing the ankle on the second pulse. Execute these motions with control, creating your own resistance and keeping your thighs and torso stationary.
- Inhale, extend the knee, and return it to the floor, with control. Thighs and torso stay stationary.
- Repeat on the left side.
- Repeat each side six to eight more times.
- Ending position: Lower your torso to the floor, into a comfortable prone position.

Knee Flexion (Femoral-on-Tibial):
Yoga Chair Pose (Utkatasana)

▶ See Fig. 14.5, Video 14.2, and Clinical Focus 14.1.
- Starting position: Standing with your legs adducted (or, for a modification, with the feet hip distance apart). Weight is centered between both feet. Arms relax by your sides.
- On an exhale, engage your core and flex your hips and knees, shifting your weight into your heels. Lower your thighs and sit back as if you were sitting on a chair. Keep your legs stationary and bring your thighs as parallel as possible to the floor while maintaining

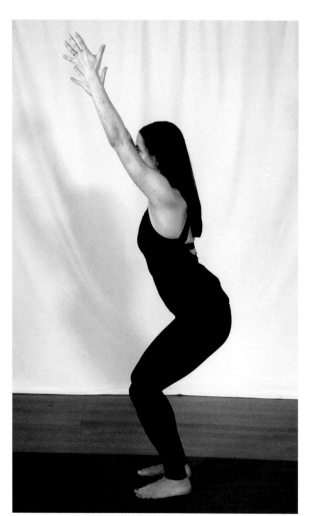

Fig. 14.5. Knee flexion (femoral-on-tibial): **Yoga Chair Pose (Utkatasana)** (see Video 14.2).

a neutral spine. (Perform the pose against a wall for extra support.)
- Inhale and flex your arms overhead, with palms facing toward each other. If this position is uncomfortable, lower your arms and join your palms together in front of your chest in a prayer position (see Video 11.3). ▶
- Keep your spine as extended as possible, with your head and neck neutral. As you flex at the hips and knees to sit deeper, lengthen from your sitting bones to the crown of your head. Ensure that your thighs are parallel to each other, the knees behind the feet and in line with the corresponding second toe.
- Maintain the position for five breath cycles.
- Ending position: On an inhale, extend your hips and knees; release your arms on the subsequent exhalation. Return to a neutral stance.

EXTENSION

If you are seated while reading this book, stand up. This requires knee (and hip) extension. Note that your upright stance is secure because extension is an intrinsically stable position; it is stable enough for you to shift your weight onto one leg and still remain erect, as when you walk. By definition, extension brings the anterior surfaces of the leg and thigh closer together. The arthrokinematics of extension are similar to those of flexion, with the movements occurring in the opposite direction. With tibial-on-femoral extension, the tibial condyles roll and slide anteriorly over the femoral condyles, moving the leg anteriorly along the sagittal plane, while the patellofemoral joint glides proximally. Try **Moving AnatoME** with the **Pilates Single Leg Kick** (see Video 14.1). Isolate ▶ tibial-on-femoral movement by keeping your thighs as stationary as possible while your knee extends.

With femoral-on-tibial extension, the femoral condyles roll anteriorly and slide posteriorly along the tibial condyles. Try **Moving AnatoME** with **Yoga Chair Pose (Utkatasana)** (see Video 14.2). As you enter into the ▶ pose, keep your legs stationary. Shift your weight into your heels and sit back as if you were sitting onto a chair, by moving only your thighs.

As with flexion, both types of full extension involve an obligatory rotation. This automatic rotation occurs at the end range of extension and produces a moderate internal rotation of the femur (in femoral-on tibial extension) or external rotation of the tibia (in tibial-on-femoral

CLINICAL FOCUS 14.1   Osteoarthritis of the Knee

Osteoarthritis is an irreversible condition characterized by progressive erosion of the hyaline cartilage lining synovial joint surfaces, such as those in the knee joint. Also called *degenerative joint disease*, osteoarthritis is caused by excessive force applied over time. For this reason, weight-bearing joints such as the knee are very susceptible, especially given how integral their movements are to our daily activities. Enter the osteoarthritic conundrum: Movement causes pain but is necessary for functionality, as well as rehabilitation. One remedy involves exercises that globally strengthen and stabilize the knee joint without involving excessive flexion, which can aggravate pain. For example, **Yoga Chair Pose** (see Video 14.2) allows individuals to isometrically strengthen their knee flexors while balancing additional muscles surrounding the knee (as well as the hip and ankle joints). Modify the degree of bend according to a pain-free range of motion; for instance, if needed, the pose may be performed with minimal flexion and/or while the back is stabilized against a wall.

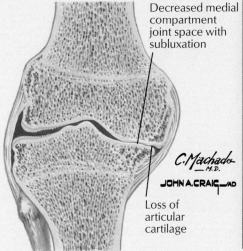

Decreased medial compartment joint space with subluxation

C. Machado M.D.
JOHN A. CRAIG—AD

Loss of articular cartilage

Knee with osteoarthritis exhibits varus deformity, medial subluxation, loss of articular cartilage, and osteophyte formation

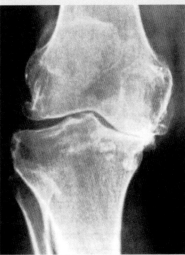

Radiograph: Varus deformity and medial subluxation of knee

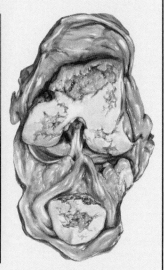

Opened knee joint. Severe erosion of articular cartilage with minimal synovial change

flexion). Often referred to as *screw-home rotation*, these biomechanics between the tibia and femur tighten ligaments and lock the fully extended knee in a stable position. Accordingly, the popliteus muscle is called "the key that unlocks the knee," because it helps bring the knee out of full extension by externally rotating the femur to initiate femoral-on-tibial flexion, or internally rotating the tibia to initiate tibial-on-femoral flexion (Practice What You Preach 14.1).

Approximate Range of Motion

5 degrees of hyperextension

PRACTICE WHAT YOU PREACH 14.1
The Busy Bee's Knees

In a standing position, the screw-home mechanism helps your knees lock to limit the amount of work needed to keep your body erect. But if you stand for too long and/or hyperextend your knees regularly—for instance, during long procedures in the operating room—aches and pains can ensue. To prevent them, perform small, balanced knee bends to gently take your knees out of a locked extension (when doing so does not interfere with the task at hand).

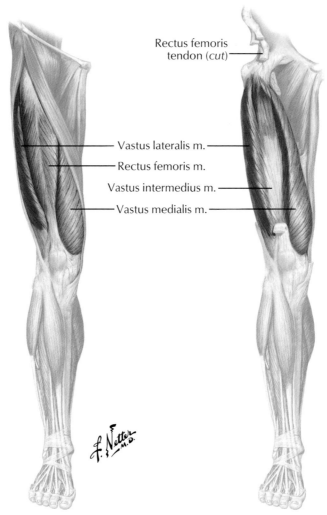

Fig. 14.6. Muscles that extend the knee.

Muscles and Innervation

See Fig. 14.6.

Muscle	Nerve
Quadriceps femoris group	
Rectus femoris	Femoral n. (L2-L4)
Vastus lateralis	Femoral n. (L2-L4)
Vastus medialis	Femoral n. (L2-L4)
Vastus intermedius	Femoral n. (L2-L4)

Moving AnatoME Exercises
Knee Extension (Tibial-on-Femoral):
Pilates Single Leg Kick

See Fig. 14.7 and Video 14.1; see **Knee Flexion (Tibial-on-Femoral)** for exercise steps.

Knee Extension (Femoral-on-Tibial):
Yoga Chair Pose (Utkatasana)

See Fig. 14.5, Video 14.2, and Clinical Focus 14.2; see **Knee Flexion (Femoral-on-Tibial)** for exercise steps.

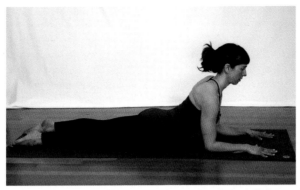

Fig. 14.7. Knee extension (tibial-on-femoral): **Pilates Single Leg Kick** (see Video 14.1).

CLINICAL FOCUS 14.2   Anterior Cruciate Ligament Tear

Large forces and regular use make the knee joint prone to abuse. We run, stretch, and jump in ways that unintentionally impact the knees and may not be aware of misuse and/or overuse until they ache, buckle, or perhaps even pop. A pop heard with a knee injury, in conjunction with other signs such as swelling and instability, is typically a sign of an anterior cruciate ligament (ACL) tear, which may be partial thickness or full thickness and may be accompanied by injury to related joint structures (eg, the meniscus or medial collateral ligament). Certain motions, such as twisting and/or hyperextension, predispose the ACL to injury, as do anatomical factors (eg, the size of the intercondylar notch and/or muscular imbalance), the female gender (women are more likely than men to incur an ACL injury in the same sport), as well as the type of surface on which an athlete plays (eg, synthetic versus natural). After an ACL injury, rest and inflammation control should be followed by rehabilitation focused on regaining range of motion, muscular balance, and strengthening core and hip musculature. Once the individual is ready to return to more regular activity, exercises such as **Pilates Single Leg Kick** (see Video 14.1) and **Yoga Chair Pose** (see Video 14.2), provide useful ways to support ongoing knee health, as they promote balanced muscular strength and proprioception.

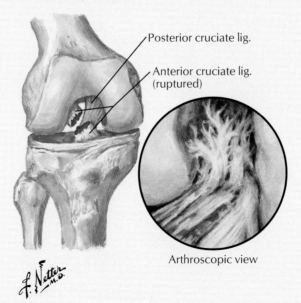

Posterior cruciate lig.

Anterior cruciate lig. (ruptured)

Arthroscopic view

BOX 14.1   **Q&A on the Q-angle**

Stand with your legs straight, feet parallel to each other, and then engage your thigh muscles to "lift" your kneecaps. Do your patellae rise in a straight line? If not—if they move laterally— you may have an increased Q-angle. The Q-angle describes the cumulative force of the quadriceps muscles relative to the knee. It is measured by two lines: a line drawn from the anterior superior iliac spine (of the pelvis) to the central patella, and a second line drawn from the central patella to the tibial tuberosity. Physicians and therapists use it to obtain information about how well the quadriceps muscles are working together and how efficiently the patella is tracking. For instance, when the Q-angle increases, so does the lateral pull on the patella during a quadriceps contraction. The vastus medialis—and, in particular, the oblique set of its fibers—is responsible for counteracting lateral pulls, i.e. from the vastus lateralis muscle. If the vastus medialis obliquus (VMO) is weak and underused, an uneven muscular contraction results, as well as misaligned patellar tracking. A properly strengthened VMO, therefore, may be key for the health of your knee and also for prevention of injury and rehabilitation following injury.

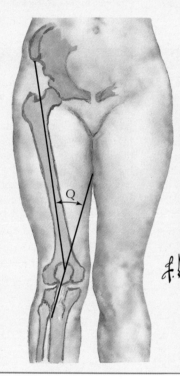

Q-angle formed by intersection of lines from anterior superior iliac spine and from tibial tuberosity through midpoint of patella. Large Q-angle predisposes to patellar subluxation.

15

Ankle

OVERVIEW

- The ankle is a hinge joint that connects the leg and foot.
- Its articulations occur between the tibia, fibula, and talus (at the talocrural joint).
- Movements include dorsiflexion and plantarflexion.
- Example exercises:
  - Dorsiflexion (**Yoga Sitting Forward Fold,** Video 15.1)
  - Plantarflexion (**Pilates Scissors,** Video 15.2)

STRUCTURE AND FUNCTION

Walking barefoot on a beach or scaling a rocky mountain requires nuanced foot placements to keep you erect. The ankle joint is one important part of this effort (Fig. 15.1). Acting as a kinetic link between the leg and foot, the ankle allows your lower limb to interact with the ground, whether you are walking, squatting, or climbing. Because it bears a lot of force (ie, the weight of your body) while you move around, its architecture endows it with a relatively high degree of stability.

The ankle joint is distal to the tibiofemoral joints, which are functionally and structurally related to the ankle. Functionally, the synovial proximal tibiofibular joint, located just below the knee, helps transfer the body's force the distal joint helps stabilize this force as it travels to the ankle. Commensurately, movement at the ankle results in slight movement at the tibiofibular joints.

Structurally, the tibiofemoral joints are comprised of the tibia and fibula bound together by the interosseous membrane, which is a sheet of connective tissue. At the most distal ends, the tibia and fibula can be prominently palpated as the "ankle bones." The distal fibula forms the lateral malleolus, and the distal tibia ends at the medial malleolus. The distal tibia and fibula are connected by strong ligaments, together forming a bracket-shaped socket into which the body of the talus projects. The talus is an important bone in the architecture of both the ankle and the foot, because it not only forms part of the ankle joint but it forms part of the subtalar and transverse tarsal joints, as well (see Chapter 16, Foot). Together, the talus, tibia, and fibula form the talocrural, or ankle, joint.

The ankle is a hinge joint surrounded by a thin capsule that is reinforced by an extensive array of collateral ligaments, such as the medial collateral (a.k.a. deltoid) ligament (see Fig. 15.1). Because of its strength (and with the help of the lateral malleolus, which forms a bony limitation to movement), the deltoid ligament limits eversion, making related sprains relatively infrequent. In contrast, the lateral collateral ligaments (including the anterior and posterior talofibular and calcaneofibular ligaments) limit inversion (see Fig. 15.1). However, they are not as strong as the deltoid ligament (plus, the medial malleolus is not as effective in providing a block as its lateral counterpart), so excessive inversion is harder to prevent and inversion sprains are more frequent (Clinical Focus 15.1).

Although eversion and inversion are well known because of the part they play in ankle sprains, they are not primary movements at the joint; rather, they occur predominately at foot joints, such as the intertarsal joints (see Chapter 16, Foot). The ankle's true movements are the hinge-like motions of dorsiflexion and plantarflexion (see Fig. 15.2). Tap your foot on the floor and observe dorsiflexion as your foot moves up and plantarflexion as your foot moves down. These ankle movements help you to not only move your foot but also to position it properly on the ground for a healthy gait.

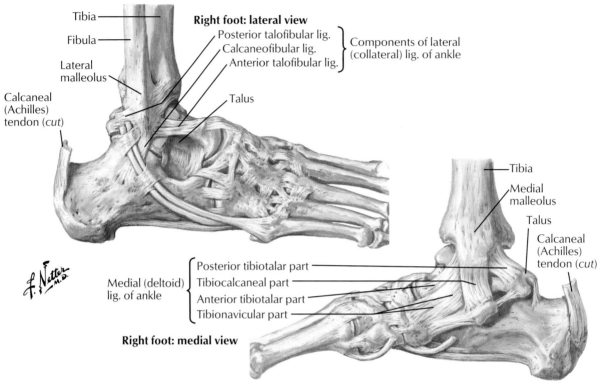

Fig. 15.1 Ankle joint.

MOVEMENT

The ankle is a synovial hinge joint. Its primary movements, dorsiflexion and plantarflexion, are necessary for everything from walking your dog, to stepping on the gas, to performing the **Yoga Tree Pose** (see Video 13.1) (Fig. 15.2). They are the "true" movements at the ankle because the joint is uniaxial, so motion occurs only along the medial-lateral axis in the sagittal plane. Other movements with which the ankle is closely associated as it functions in conjunction with the foot complex (eg, eversion, inversion, abduction, adduction, pronation, and supination) are discussed in Chapter 16, The Foot, along with the primary joints responsible for the movements (eg, subtalar and transverse tarsal joints). Together, the ankle and foot complex acts as a kinetic linkage that allows the lower limbs to interface with the ground.

DORSIFLEXION

Each time you place your heel on the ground to take a step forward, you rely on dorsiflexion of your foot, which brings the dorsum of the foot closer to the anterior leg. Dorsiflexion occurs as the superior surface of the talus rolls and slides posteriorly along the combined tibial-fibular articulating surface when the foot is in an open chain position (eg, during the swing phase of walking). Much of the time, however, the foot dorsiflexes in a closed chain position, as seen during the stance phase of walking. In this case, the tibial-fibular surface rolls and slides anteriorly along the talus. Ligaments that become taught (eg, calcaneofibular ligament) limit the extent of the posterior slide and, hence, dorsiflexion. Because the anterior portion of the talus, which is wider than the posterior portion, connects with the tibia and fibula, the articulation is inherently tight. Dorsiflexion is thereby a stable position for the ankle and foot, which makes sense, given that it is a basic part of bipedal stance and locomotion. Of note, dorsiflexion of the entire foot occurs in conjunction with movement at many of the joints of the foot, such as the transverse tarsal and tarsometatarsal joints (see Chapter 16, Foot). Try **Moving AnatoME** with **Yoga Sitting Forward Fold (Paschimottanasana)** (see Video 15.1). After you have entered the pose, see if you

CLINICAL FOCUS 15.1   Ankle Sprains

You are strolling along the sidewalk when, suddenly, your foot slips on cracked pavement. Your ankle twists, your foot inverts, and when you try to bear weight, your ankle hurts. Most likely, you injured one or more of your ankle ligaments. Even though inversion primarily occurs at the subtalar joint of the foot, the ankle is a weaker joint and, hence, more susceptible to injury. Also, inversion (along with plantarflexion) is an inherently unstable position and therefore a common mechanism of sprains. Inversion sprains typically involve damage to the lateral ligaments of the ankle joint, with the anterior talofibular ligament most likely to be injured (because it is the least elastic of the lateral ligaments). Repeat sprains, however, may be due to a variety of reasons including abnormal proprioception, and improperly healed ligaments from previous strains. Whether one is rebounding from an acute or a chronic injury, early mobility is preferred over immobility; full stability may take months to regain, however. One way to ease into ankle motion is the **Seated Foot Strengthening exercise** (see Video 16.1), which provides an introduction to ankle and foot movements and also strengthens the fibular muscles, which help prevent excessive inversion.

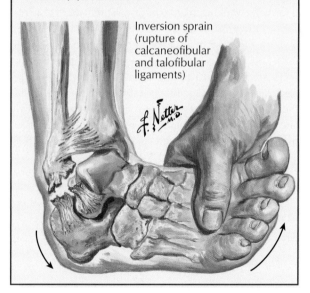

Inversion sprain (rupture of calcaneofibular and talofibular ligaments)

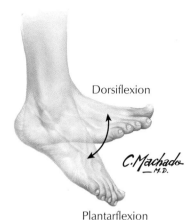

Fig. 15.2 Ankle movements.

can dorsiflex your feet a bit more but without gripping the thigh muscles.

Approximate Range of Motion

20 degrees; the amount of dorsiflexion necessary to walk is about 10 degrees

Muscles and Innervation

See Fig. 15.3.

Muscle	Nerve
Tibialis anterior	Deep peroneal n. (L4, L5)
Extensor digitorum longus	Deep peroneal n. (L5, S1)
Extensor hallucis longus	Deep peroneal n. (L5, S1)
Fibularis tertius	Deep peroneal n. (L5, S1)

Moving AnatoME Exercise

Ankle Dorsiflexion: Yoga Sitting Forward Fold (Paschimottanasana)

See Fig. 15.4 and Video 15.1.

- Starting position: Sitting on the floor with legs extended and adducted in front of you, feet dorsiflexed. If you need help maintaining an erect torso, place a cushion under your pelvis. Arms are by your sides with palms pressing into the ground.
- Keeping your spine as neutral as possible, flex forward at your hips. This movement will bring your chest toward your shins.

Superficial dissection   **Deep dissection**

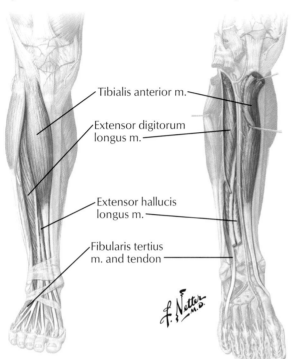

Tibialis anterior m.

Extensor digitorum longus m.

Extensor hallucis longus m.

Fibularis tertius m. and tendon

Fig. 15.3 Muscles that dorsiflex the ankle.

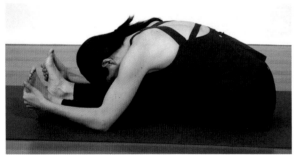

Fig. 15.4 Ankle dorsiflexion: **Yoga Sitting Forward Fold (Paschimottanasana)** (see Video 15.1).

• As you hinge forward, grasp the lateral edges of your feet with your hands; if this is not possible, place your hands either on your shins or on the floor beside them. Keep dorsiflexing the feet and extending the toes, reaching through your heels.

• At the extent of the stretch, gently flex forward through your vertebral column and head. It should feel like a release.
• Remain for five slow breaths, folding deeper on each exhale.
• Ending position: On an inhale, extend your vertebral column into a neutral position and return it to the upright starting position.

PLANTARFLEXION

Every time you "put the pedal to the metal" in your car (ie, step on the gas), you are plantarflexing your foot. The reverse of dorsiflexion, plantarflexion brings the plantar aspect (eg, sole) of the foot closer to the posterior leg. In an open chain position, it occurs when the trochlear surface of the talus rolls and slides anteriorly in the combined curvature of the tibia and fibula, loosening most of the collateral ligaments surrounding the joint. This loosening, especially when weight bearing, makes plantarflexion a less stable position than dorsiflexion. Nonetheless, plantarflexion is equally important for bipedalism; for example, after the heel of your right foot contacts the floor while walking, plantarflexion rapidly lowers the rest of it to the ground for a brief stance, which is followed by push-off. As with dorsiflexion, when plantarflexion of the whole foot is occurring, many of the joints of the foot (eg, transverse tarsal and tarsometatarsal joints) also play a role (see Chapter 16, Foot). Try **Moving AnatoME** with the **Pilates Scissors** (see Video 15.2). Plantarflex slowly and see if you can isolate the movement (eg, without pronation or supination) (Practice What You Preach 15.1).

Approximate Range of Motion
60 degrees

Muscles and Innervation
See Figs. 15.5 and 14.3.

Muscle	Nerve
Gastrocnemius	Tibial n. (S1, S2)
Soleus	Tibial n. (S1, S2)
Plantaris	Tibial n. (S1, S2)
Tibialis posterior	Tibial n. (L4, L5)
Flexor digitorum longus	Tibial n. (S2, S3)
Flexor hallucis longus	Tibial n. (S2, S3)
Fibularis longus	Superficial fibular n. (L5-S2)
Fibularis brevis	Superficial fibular n. (L5-S2)

PRACTICE WHAT YOU PREACH 15.1
High Heels, High Cost

High-heeled shoes can cost a lot in the store, and they can also have a cost for your body. By shifting the body's weight over a plantarflexed ankle, these shoes place the talocrural joint in an unstable position. This position loosens the tibial and fibular encapsulation of the talus and slackens most of the collateral ligaments and plantarflexor muscles. These changes shift one's posture, causing ripple effects on the joints, ligaments, and muscles from feet to head. If you need to wear heels, take them off at regular intervals to give your body a break. You can also perform ankle circles in each direction, to relieve pressure and move each ankle through its full range of motion.

Moving AnatoME Exercise
Ankle Plantarflexion: Pilates Scissors
See Fig. 15.6 and Video 15.2.

- Starting position: Lying supine with your pelvis in a posterior tilt (see Video 13.2). Your hips are flexed to 90 degrees, with legs extended, and ankles, feet, and toes are plantarflexed. Arms are by your sides with palms on the floor.
- Inhale to prepare.
- Exhale, and nod your chin toward your chest as you gently flex your head, neck, and thoracic spine off the floor, reaching your hands to grasp your right leg as you "scissor" your legs apart (flexing your right hip to bring the right thigh closer to your torso and extending your left hip so that your left thigh hovers above the ground). Perform the exhale in two staccato pulses.

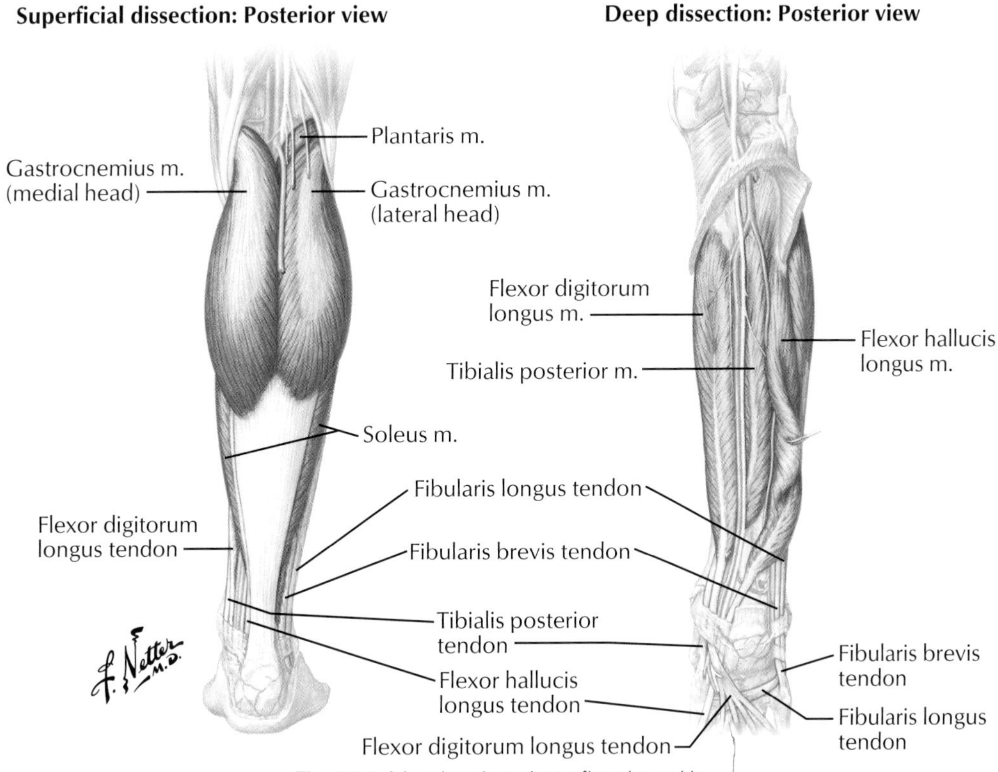

Superficial dissection: Posterior view   **Deep dissection: Posterior view**

Plantaris m.

Gastrocnemius m. (medial head)

Gastrocnemius m. (lateral head)

Flexor digitorum longus m.

Tibialis posterior m.

Flexor hallucis longus m.

Soleus m.

Flexor digitorum longus tendon

Fibularis longus tendon

Fibularis brevis tendon

Tibialis posterior tendon

Flexor hallucis longus tendon

Fibularis brevis tendon

Fibularis longus tendon

Flexor digitorum longus tendon

Fig. 15.5 Muscles that plantarflex the ankle.

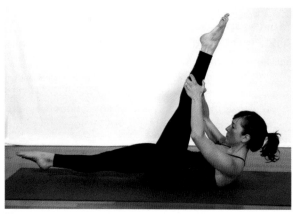

Fig. 15.6 Ankle plantarflexion: **Pilates Scissors** (see Video 15.2).

- Inhale to scissor. Switch legs as you extend your right hip so that the right thigh hovers above the ground, and flex the left hip to bring the left thigh closer to the torso.
- Exhale as you grasp the left leg and pulse twice.
- While scissoring, keep plantarflexing through each ankle, creating a sense of length through the lower extremities. Engage your core to maintain a stable torso and prevent rotation of the spine and pelvis.
- Repeat each side six to eight times.
- Ending position: Slowly lower your arms, legs, and torso to the floor.

16

Foot

OVERVIEW

- The foot is the region distal to the leg. It is composed of 28 bones, which form the rearfoot (talus and calcaneus), midfoot (remaining tarsal bones), and forefoot (metatarsals, phalanges, and sesamoids).
- Articulations occur between the talus, calcaneus, and tarsal bones (intertarsal joints), the tarsal and metatarsal bones (tarsometatarsal joints), the metatarsal bones and phalanges (metatarsophalangeal joints), and the phalanges (interphalangeal joints).
- Movements include:
  - Foot: dorsiflexion, plantarflexion, abduction, adduction, eversion, inversion, pronation, and supination.
  - Toes: flexion, extension, abduction, and adduction.
- Example exercises:
  - Dorsiflexion (**Yoga Sitting Forward Fold,** Video 15.1)
  - Plantarflexion (**Pilates Scissors,** Video 15.2)
  - Abduction (**Seated Foot Strengthening,** Video 16.1)
  - Adduction (**Seated Foot Strengthening,** Video 16.1)
  - Eversion (**Yoga Half Lord of the Fishes Pose,** (Video 16.2)
  - Inversion (**Pilates Seal,** Video 16.3)

STRUCTURE AND FUNCTION

Although you likely pay little attention to your feet, one quarter of your body's bones reside there. These bones, and the ligaments that connect them, form a well-designed foundation for the rest of your body. Indeed, some researchers have found that these bones, along with the surrounding connective tissue, form a structure that is strong enough to support you in an ideal standing position; in other words, a passive stance on healthy feet requires little or no activity of the foot muscles. Your bipedal stance, whether ideal or not, is a hallmark of *Homo sapiens*, one that allows you to use your hands to interact with your environment as your feet transport you from place to place.

Each foot thereby supports both posture and locomotion. This dual functionality came about after evolution changed the more muscular structure of our primate brethren to the group of ligament-bound bones we see today in the human body. There are 28 bones in each foot and ankle (including the two sesamoids located within the tendon of the flexor hallucis brevis muscle). In the body, wherever there are lots of bones (eg, in the hand), there are lots of joints, and, hence, lots of movements are available. Multiple movements allow your feet to safely traverse many types of terrain (eg, rocky or sandy). The thousands of nerve endings in the plantar surface, or sole, of the foot make this surface one of the most sensitive areas of skin on your body. This sensitivity helps in a variety of ways, from getting you off hot sand, to preventing falls, to deciding where and how to place your foot with each step (proprioception).

Four primary sets of joints are responsible for the movements of your foot and toes: intertarsal (IT), tarsometatarsal (TMT), metatarsophalangeal (MTP), and interphalangeal (IP) joints. Although this classification of joints resembles that of the hand, there is one big difference: Unlike the thumb, the great toe is in line with the other digits of the foot and structurally bound to them via the transverse metatarsal ligament. This arrangement adapts the foot for stability, propulsion, and weight bearing, but it prevents opposability (as seen with the thumb), limiting the great toe's, and, hence, the foot's, range of motion in comparison with that of the thumb and hand (Fig. 16.1).

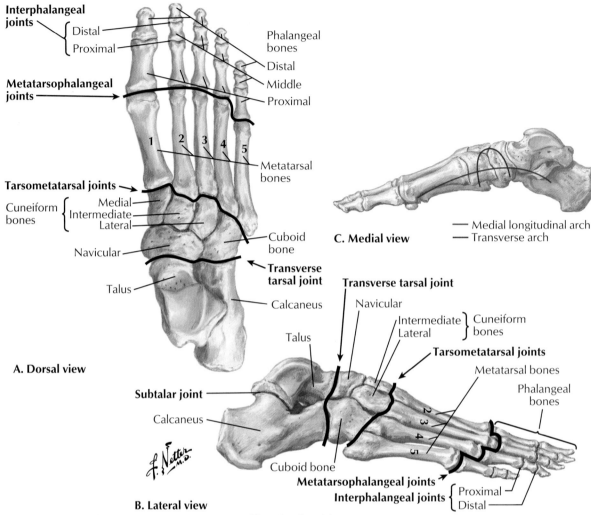

Interphalangeal joints
{ Distal
  Proximal }

Metatarsophalangeal joints

Phalangeal bones
- Distal
- Middle
- Proximal

Metatarsal bones
1 2 3 4 5

Tarsometatarsal joints

Cuneiform bones {
  Medial
  Intermediate
  Lateral }

Navicular

Talus

Cuboid bone

Transverse tarsal joint

Calcaneus

A. Dorsal view

Subtalar joint

Calcaneus

Cuboid bone

B. Lateral view

Transverse tarsal joint

Navicular

Intermediate } Cuneiform
Lateral   } bones

Tarsometatarsal joints

Metatarsal bones

Phalangeal bones

Talus

2 3 4 5

Metatarsophalangeal joints
Interphalangeal joints { Proximal
                             Distal }

C. Medial view
— Medial longitudinal arch
— Transverse arch

f. Netter M.D.

Fig. 16.1 Foot joints.

Intertarsal Joints

The tarsal bones, which are organized into proximal and distal rows, include the talus, calcaneus, navicular bone, cuneiform bones (medial, intermediate, and lateral), and cuboid bone. The articulations between these seven bones form the intertarsal (IT) joints, which can be further categorized into subtalar and transverse tarsal joints. The subtalar joint is the set of articulations formed between the calcaneus and talus, in the rearfoot. When the bones slide and rotate upon each other, they facilitate eversion, inversion, abduction, and adduction; the movements are typically coupled, with eversion and abduction occurring together and inversion and adduction occurring together. The calcaneus can also dorsiflex and plantarflex relative

to the talus, but the movements are small in and of themselves and even more so relative to the range of the ankle joint. Typically, the joint movements are referenced in terms of a mobile calcaneus against a fixed talus, but the reverse also happens (ie, during the stance phase of walking, when the calcaneus is relatively immobile). Overall, subtalar joint mobility allows your foot to assume positions that are independent of leg placement; for example, if you step on a rock while walking, your foot can evert to accommodate the terrain while your leg, along with the rest of you, remains vertical.

The transverse tarsal joint, in turn, consists of the talonavicular joint (between the talus and navicular bone), as well as the calcaneocuboid joint (between the calcaneus and cuboid bones). Its composite joint structure is located in the midfoot and stabilized by the medial longitudinal arch, specialized ligaments, and its joint capsule. Joint mobility allows for dorsiflexion and plantarflexion, abduction and adduction, and inversion and eversion. They tend to occur in combination, for example, abduction occurs with dorsiflexion and adduction occurs with plantarflexion. Also, although the transverse tarsal joint has its own form of movement, it rarely functions without the subtalar joint. Together, these joints enable most of the foot's motions of pronation and supination; they are assisted by distal IT joints (ie, cuneonavicular, cuboideonavicular) that also function to stabilize the foot by forming its transverse arch.

Tarsometatarsal Joints

As with the metacarpal bones of the hand, you have five metatarsal bones in each foot. They are distal to the tarsal bones, mentioned above, and form five articulations: first metatarsal and medial cuneiform, second metatarsal and intermediate cuneiform, third metatarsal and lateral cuneiform, fourth metatarsal and cuboid, and fifth metatarsal and cuboid. Working together, these tarsometatarsal (TMT) joints enable primarily dorsiflexion and plantarflexion, combined with eversion and inversion. Mobility tends to be greatest at the more lateral joints; TMT mobility may be augmented by some motion at the intermetatarsal joints found at the bases of the four lateral metatarsals.

Metatarsophalangeal Joints

Each of the five metatarsal bones articulates with a proximal phalanx. Although they are small, each synovial joint includes articular cartilage, ligaments, and a fibrous capsule. These metatarsophalangeal (MTP) joints of the forefoot coordinate to move the foot and toes through flexion, extension, abduction, and adduction. Spread your toes to observe that abduction and adduction tend to be the more limited of the movements (Practice What You Preach 16.1).

Interphalangeal Joints

Your foot has five phalanges, or toes. Each toe has a proximal, middle, and distal phalanx, with the exception of the big toe, which, like the thumb, lacks a middle bone. The articulation between two adjacent phalanges forms an interphalangeal (IP) joint (Latin *inter*, "between" and *phalanx*, "row of soldiers"). These joints move the toes through flexion and extension. Your toes have a smaller range of extension (compared to flexion), as

---

PRACTICE WHAT YOU PREACH 16.1
Big Toe Bunions

Although a bunion (hallux vlagus) appears as a superficial red bump on the medial aspect of the big toe, the problem is deeper. A bunion involves a medial deviation at your first metatarsal head, with a lateral deviation of your big toe (hallux). Whether the bunion is caused by genetics, joint structure, incorrect footwear, or pronated or flat feet, it may cause pain whether standing or walking. To manage bunion pain, wear shoes that are large enough for the bump and for wiggling your toes. You can also take several seconds to gently hold your big toe in alignment. It might not make the bunion disappear, but it will promote greater mobility and comfort.

---

the movement is limited by the toe flexor muscles and ligaments found in the sole of the foot. The joints are subdivided as proximal interphalangeal (PIP) and distal interphalangeal (DIP) joints.

Summary

Each set of joints contributes to multiple foot movements (Fig. 16.2). In many cases, it is difficult to isolate a movement at a specific joint (eg, transverse tarsal and subtalar movements) or to isolate movements from each other (eg, abduction and dorsiflexion at the transverse tarsal joint). The joints and movements are detailed here to provide an introductory sense of the foot's complexity and the resulting level of nuanced movement available. As with the shoulder joint, however, it is important to keep in mind the big picture while learning the details.

MOVEMENT

The foot's intrinsic articulations, at the IT, TMT, MTP, and IP joints, enable movement in a number of ways (eg, running, skipping, and prancing) and on a variety of surfaces (eg, steep, bumpy, or slippery) (Fig. 16.2). Recall, also, that the ankle joint moves the foot, primarily through dorsiflexion and plantarflexion; it is described separately for structural purposes (see Chapter 15, Ankle). Together, the ankle and foot joints function as a complex that permits triplanar movement of the foot and toes. Muscles that are both intrinsic (found within the foot) and extrinsic (arising from the leg) enable the movements, which include dorsiflexion, plantarflexion, abduction, adduction, as well as eversion and inversion, which occur solely at the foot. The foot is also able to pronate and supinate; these are compound movements (similar to

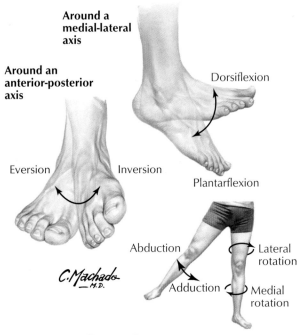

Around a medial-lateral axis

Around an anterior-posterior axis

Dorsiflexion

Eversion   Inversion

Plantarflexion

C. Machado —M.D.

Abduction   Adduction   Lateral rotation   Medial rotation

Fig. 16.2 Foot movements.

BOX 16.1   The Weight of the World

As your most distal appendages, your feet carry the entire load of your body whether you are skipping or salsa dancing. In large part, this facility is due to the support and shock-absorbing properties of the medial longitudinal arch. One of three arches (the others are the lateral and transverse arches), the medial longitudinal arch is composed of the calcaneus, talus, navicular bone, cuneiforms, and metatarsals 1 to 3 and it is supported by the plantar fascia (see Clinical Focus 16.1). When standing, the architecture of this arch—along with surrounding connective tissue—should be strong enough to keep you upright without active muscle involvement. Without this arch, the force that your foot incurs while you are sprinting, for example, would likely exceed the weight-bearing capacity of your foot bones, alone. Stress is further mitigated as the arch disperses the force evenly throughout your foot so it can move healthily up the biomechanical chain of your lower extremity. Further assisting the arch is the first TMT joint, which offers an element of flexibility as it slightly dorsiflexes under your body's weight (see Practice What You Preach 16.2).

circumduction of the shoulder and opposition of the thumb). Pronation includes elements of eversion, abduction, and dorsiflexion; supination includes elements of inversion, adduction, and plantarflexion (Box 16.1).

DORSIFLEXION

When you tie your shoelaces, you lift the top of your foot toward you (while your heel remains on the floor). Dorsiflexion brings the dorsum of the foot closer to the anterior leg. Most of the foot's ability to dorsiflex arises at the ankle joint; for further information, see Chapter 15, Ankle. The remainder of the ability to dorsiflex occurs at the foot's intrinsic joints, primarily at the combined transverse tarsal and subtalar joints. The TMT joints also assist dorsiflexion.

Many times, when you dorsiflex your foot you also extend your toes. The toes are extended every time you lift them off the ground—or when you lift yourself, as when you're "standing on your tiptoes." This extension, particularly at the big toe, is necessary for push-off with every step you take forward. The movement occurs primarily at the MTP joints in a sagittal plane about a medial-lateral axis. It also occurs at the uniaxial IP joints, although the movement is limited due to the presence

of the toe flexor muscles, as well as the plantar ligaments. Try **Moving AnatoME** with the **Yoga Sitting Forward Fold (Paschimottanasana)** (see Video 15.1), and note how you can extend your toes farther than your foot.

Approximate Range of Motion

TMT: Minimal
MTP: Lateral four toes, 65 degrees; big toe, 85 degrees
PIP and DIP: 30 degrees

Muscles and Innervation

See Fig. 16.3 (see Fig. 16.4 for lumbricals). See Chapter 15, Ankle, for muscles that dorsiflex the foot.

Muscle	Nerve
Extensor digitorum longus	Deep peroneal n. (L5, S1)
Extensor hallucis longus	Deep peroneal n. (L5, S1)
Extensor digitorum brevis	Deep peroneal n. (L5, S1)
Lumbricals, at IP joints	Lateral three: lateral plantar n. (S2, S3) Medial one: medial plantar n. (S2, S3)

CLINICAL FOCUS 16.1   Plantar Fasciitis

The plantar fascia on the sole of your foot is a thick connective tissue that acts as a shock absorber, in part by providing tension and elasticity for the medial longitudinal arch. When the plantar fascia is weakened or overstretched, therefore, it cannot properly support the arch or the body's weight (and it then requires compensation by the extrinsic and intrinsic foot muscles); muscular imbalances, like a tight calcaneal tendon, can also negatively impact the fascia. Weakening may occur when excess weight and/or tension is placed on the arch, as occurs with obesity, during pregnancy, or when one endures repetitive stress (eg, when running), has poor shoe support, and/or is affected by anatomical variations such as pes planus. Irritation and inflammation may occur as greater demands are placed on the fascia than it can handle, leading to

plantar fasciitis. Symptoms of this condition typically include heel pain felt medially, pain that is felt in the morning and worsens with activity, and tenderness to palpation. Many individuals are unaware of the plantar fascia until it hurts. To prevent or rehabilitate plantar fasciitiis, stretching the fascia is recommended. A convenient stretch involves sitting in a chair, cross-legged, resting the affected foot atop the contralateral thigh. Grasp the forefoot (just distal to the MTP joints), manually extending the toes until a stretch in the arch is felt. Hold the stretch for at least 10 seconds, relax the foot, and repeat up to three times. To know that you are stretching the proper area, palpate the tension in the plantar fascia with the contralateral hand while performing the stretch.

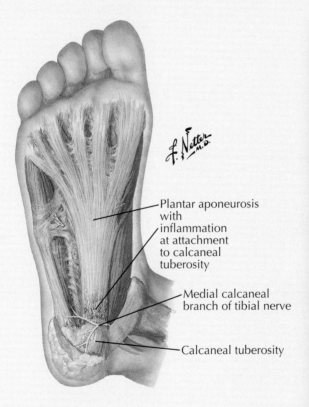

Plantar aponeurosis with inflammation at attachment to calcaneal tuberosity

Medial calcaneal branch of tibial nerve

Calcaneal tuberosity

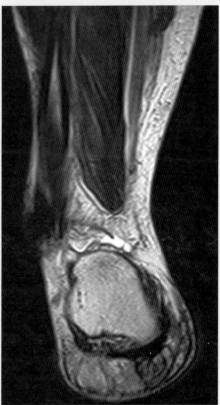

Plantar fasciitis as shown on magnetic resonance imaging (MRI)

Moving AnatoME Exercise

Foot Dorsiflexion: Yoga Sitting Forward Fold (Paschimottanasana)

See Fig. 15.4 and Video 15.1.

PLANTARFLEXION

When a ballerina points her foot to create a graceful, continuous line with her leg, she is plantarflexing. Plantarflexion brings the plantar aspect (a.k.a. sole) of the foot closer to the posterior leg. Most of the foot's ability to plantarflex arises at the ankle joint; for further information, see Chapter 15, Ankle. Further plantarflexion occurs within the foot, at the transverse tarsal and subtalar joints. The TMT joints additionally assist plantarflexion.

Most of the time, when you plantarflex your foot, you concurrently flex your toes. Toe flexion is experienced,

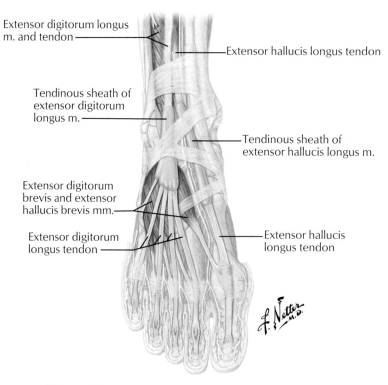

Fig. 16.3 Muscles that dorsiflex the foot and extend the toes.

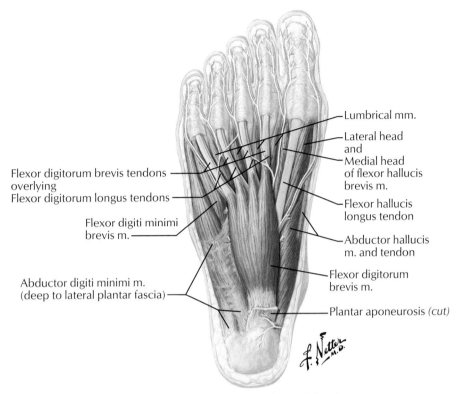

Lumbrical mm.

Lateral head and Medial head of flexor hallucis brevis m.

Flexor digitorum brevis tendons overlying

Flexor digitorum longus tendons

Flexor hallucis longus tendon

Flexor digiti minimi brevis m.

Abductor hallucis m. and tendon

Flexor digitorum brevis m.

Abductor digiti minimi m. (deep to lateral plantar fascia)

Plantar aponeurosis *(cut)*

Fig. 16.4 Muscles that plantarflex the foot and flex the toes.

for example, when you grip your toes while walking in flip-flops, in order to keep them on. As with extension, flexion occurs at the MTP joints in a sagittal plane about a medial-lateral axis, as well as at the uniaxial IP joints. Toe flexion helps your body both adapt to its substrate and remain balanced upon it, as evidenced when walking a tightrope. Try **Moving AnatoME** with **Pilates Scissors** (see Video 15.2), and note how your toes continue the line of flexion of the foot (similarly, for example, to how the neck extension in the **Yoga Cobra Pose** [see Video 6.2] is a natural continuation of the rest of your spine).

Approximate Range of Motion

TMT: Minimal
MTP: 30 degrees
PIP and DIP: 70 degrees

Muscles and Innervation

See Fig. 16.4 (see Fig. 16.7 for adductor hallucis muscle). See Chapter 15, Ankle, for muscles that plantarflex the foot.

Muscle	Nerve
Flexor digitorum longus	Tibial n. (S2, S3)
Flexor hallucis longus	Tibial n. (S2, S3)
Flexor digitorum brevis	Medial plantar n. (S2, S3)
Flexor hallucis brevis	Medial plantar n. (S2, S3)
Flexor digiti minimi	Superficial branch of lateral plantar n.
Abductor digiti minimi	Lateral plantar n. (S2, S3)
Abductor hallucis	Medial plantar n. (S2, S3)
Adductor hallucis	Deep branch of lateral plantar n. (S2, S3)
Lumbricals, at MTP joints	Lateral three: lateral plantar n. (S2, S3) Medial one: medial plantar n. (S2, S3)

Moving AnatoME Exercise

Foot Plantarflexion: Pilates Scissors

See Fig. 15.6 and Video 15.2.

ABDUCTION

The Charleston dance of the 1920s was renowned for flappers swiveling their feet in and out as they stepped forward and back. Swiveling of the foot outward, which turns the foot away from the midline, involves abduction (which, in that dance form, appears exaggerated by virtue of concurrent external rotation at the hip joint). Abduction occurs at the subtalar joint; the movement is aided by the transverse tarsal joint. Abduction helps you adjust to the terrain on which you are walking and, in that situation, typically happens in conjunction with eversion.

The toes are also able to abduct. When you "spread your toes on your yoga mat," for example, you are abducting them. Toe abduction occurs at the MTP joints in the horizontal plane about a vertical axis. Try **Moving AnatoMe** with the **Seated Foot Strengthening** exercise (see Video 16.1) to isolate and strengthen your foot abductors. Foot abduction is a very subtle movement; after you do it, separately practice abducting your toes. For resistance, use a resistance band, pillowcase, or thin towel.

Approximate Range of Motion

MTP: Difficult to measure independently
IT: 15 degrees at subtalar joint

Muscles and Innervation

See Fig. 16.5. See Chapter 15, Ankle, for muscles that abduct the foot.

Muscle	Nerve
Abductor hallucis	Medial plantar n. (S2, S3)
Abductor digiti minimi	Lateral plantar n. (S2, S3)
Flexor digitorum brevis	Medial plantar n. (S2, S3)
Dorsal interossei	Lateral plantar n. (S2, S3)

Moving AnatoME Exercise
Foot Abduction: Seated Foot Strengthening

See Fig. 16.6 and Video 16.1.
- Starting position: Sitting on the floor with a resistance band (or towel). Legs are extended in front of you, feet are dorsiflexed. If you need help maintaining an

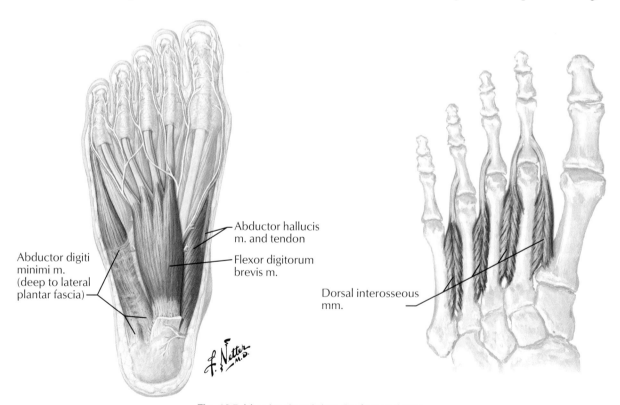

Fig. 16.5 Muscles that abduct the foot and toes.

Abductor hallucis m. and tendon

Flexor digitorum brevis m.

Abductor digiti minimi m. (deep to lateral plantar fascia)

Dorsal interosseous mm.

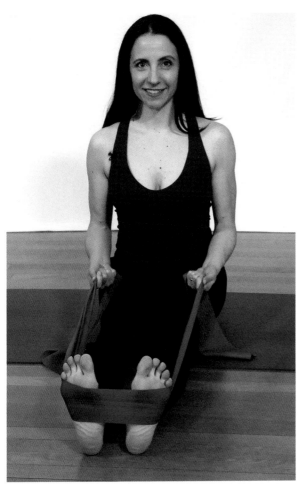

Fig. 16.6 Foot abduction: **Seated Foot Strengthening** (see Video 16.1).

erect torso, place a cushion under your pelvis. Arms are by your sides with palms pressing into the ground.

- Keep your thighs parallel and dorsiflex your feet, reaching actively through the heels and extending the toes.
- Hold each end of the resistance band and wrap it around the balls of your feet. Then, return your torso to an upright position.
- Maintaining dorsiflexion, slowly abduct your feet so that your toes angle outward. Isolate the movement at the foot joints (versus externally rotating the hips). The degree of movement is minimal.

- Return your feet to a neutral position and repeat four more times. Make sure that your weight remains even on your sitting bones, with the torso elongated.
- Similarly adduct your feet four times. This range of movement is also minimal.
- As an addition to the exercise, you can abduct and adduct the toes as you move the feet, respectively.
- Ending position: Release the band and relax your feet, sitting with legs extended.

ADDUCTION

In the description of abduction, the Charleston dance of the 1920s was mentioned as an example. The dance illustrates adduction as well, when the flapper swivels her feet inward. This inward foot swivel, which turns the toes toward the midline, involves adduction (and, in that dance form, appears exaggerated by virtue of internal rotation at the hip joint). Like abduction, adduction occurs primarily at the subtalar joint, as the calcaneus rotates about a fixed talus (or vice versa); it is aided by the transverse tarsal joint. While it is possible (though challenging) to isolate the motions as separate movements, adduction typically happens in conjunction with inversion.

The toes are also able to adduct, as when you squeeze them together to fit into pointy shoes. This movement occurs at the MTP joints in the horizontal plane about a vertical axis. Try **Moving AnatoMe** with **Seated Foot Strengthening** exercise (see Video 16.1) to isolate and strengthen your foot adductors. Foot adduction is a very subtle movement; after you do it, separately practice adducting your toes. For resistance, use a resistance band, pillowcase, or thin towel.

Approximate Range of Motion

MTP: limited and difficult to measure independently
IT: 30 degrees at subtalar joint

Muscles and Innervation

See Fig. 16.7 (see Fig. 16.10 for the tibialis anterior muscle).

Muscle	Nerve
Adductor hallucis	Deep branch of lateral plantar n. (S2, S3)
Plantar interossei	Lateral plantar n. (S2, S3)
Tibialis anterior	Deep fibular n. (L4, L5)

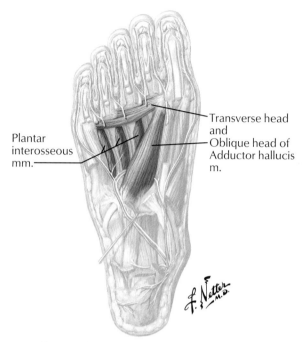

Plantar interosseous mm.

Transverse head and Oblique head of Adductor hallucis m.

Fig. 16.7 Muscles that adduct the foot and toes.

Moving AnatoME Exercise
Foot Adduction: Seated Foot Strengthening

See Fig. 16.8 and Video 16.1; see **Abduction** for exercise steps.

EVERSION

Sitting in your chair, rotate your left foot so that its sole points outward. This movement is eversion, which turns the plantar aspect of the foot away from the midline. Eversion is a relatively small movement, and not one that is intentionally isolated on a regular basis. Nonetheless, you evert your foot throughout the day as the movement helps your foot adapt to uneven ground. To evert, the subtalar joint moves as the calcaneus rotates medially about a fixed talus, as when stepping on a rock with the lateral side of your foot (causing the medial side to fall to the ground). The movement can also occur with the talus rotating laterally around a fixed calcaneus (eg, when "cutting" to change directions during a soccer game). Eversion at the subtalar joint is assisted by the transverse tarsal and TMT joints. Try **Moving AnatoMe** with the **Yoga Half Lord of the Fishes Pose (Ardha Matsyen-drasana)** (see Video 16.2). As you prepare your seated

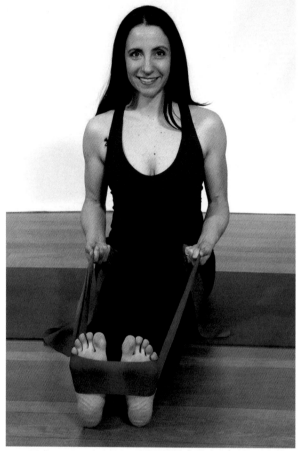

Fig. 16.8 Foot adduction: **Seated Foot Strengthening** (see Video 16.1).

foundation, notice how you will likely need to evert your top foot in order to place the entire plantar surface of the foot on the ground.

Approximate Range of Motion
12 degrees

Muscles and Innervation
See Fig. 16.9.

Muscle	Nerve
Fibularis longus	Superficial fibular n. (L5-S2)
Fibularis brevis	Superficial fibular n. (L5-S2)
Fibularis tertius	Superficial fibular n. (L5, S1)
Extensor digitorum longus	Deep fibular n. (L5, S1)

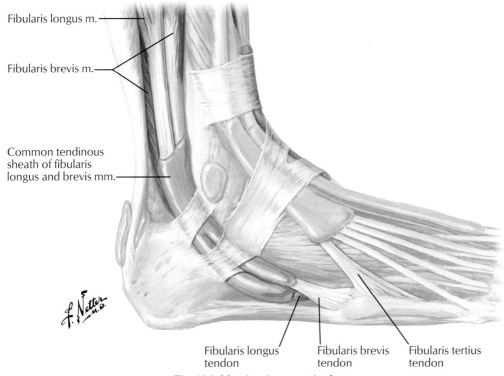

Fibularis longus m.—

Fibularis brevis m.—

Common tendinous
sheath of fibularis
longus and brevis mm.—

Fibularis longus
tendon

Fibularis brevis
tendon

Fibularis tertius
tendon

Fig. 16.9 Muscles that evert the foot.

Moving AnatoME Exercise

Foot Eversion: Yoga Half Lord of the Fishes Pose
(Ardha Matsyendrasana)

See Fig. 16.10 and Video 16.2.

- Starting position: Sitting on the floor with legs extended in front of you, feet dorsiflexed. If you need help maintaining an erect torso, place a cushion under your pelvis. Arms are by your sides with palms pressing into the floor.
- Engage your core, flex your knees, and slide your left foot under the right leg to place it outside of the right ischial tuberosity (sitting bone). Then cross your right leg over the left, placing the right foot by the outside of the left knee. Evert the right foot to place the entire plantar surface of the right foot on the floor. Your right knee points toward the ceiling. Make sure your weight is even on your sitting bones.
- Inhale and abduct your left arm to 180 degrees, as you extend your spine and place your right hand behind you, gently pressing your right fingertips into the ground to help lengthen the spine. Exhale and rotate your torso toward the right thigh, wrapping

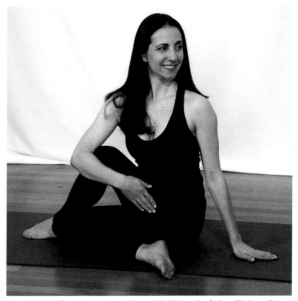

Fig. 16.10 Foot eversion: **Yoga Half Lord of the Fishes Pose (Ardha Matsyendrasana)** (see Video 16.2).

your left arm around your right knee. Keep extending and rotating the spine, bringing the anterior torso and right thigh as close together as possible.

- Rotate your head to the right, and gaze diagonally toward the back wall.
- In the pose, maintain eversion of the right foot to keep its plantar surface in contact with the floor. Keep your chest open and broad. On each inhale, lengthen your torso. On each exhale, rotate it slightly more to the right.
- Remain here for five breaths.
- Reverse sides.
- Ending position: On an exhale, rotate your torso back to face the front, release your arms to your sides, and bring your legs into a comfortable cross-legged position.

Of note, most yoga and Pilates movements do not evert intentionally, because (1) the durable deltoid ligament on the medial side of the ankle prevents excess movement and (2) eversion is not a very stable position.

INVERSION

Because inversion is a generally unstable position, you most often use it during a movement class when you are counteracting a tendency to evert. For instance, if your back foot's lateral edge tends to lift off the ground during the **Yoga Warrior II Pose (Virabhadrasana II)** (see Video 13.8), inversion restores your foot to a balanced position. Inversion brings the plantar aspect of your foot toward the midline. It is the counterpart to eversion, likewise occurring at the subtalar joint, and assisted by the transverse tarsal and TMT joints. When inverting, the calcaneus rotates laterally relative to a fixed talus, as when you step on a rock with the medial side of your foot (causing the lateral side to fall toward the ground). Try **Moving AnatoMe** with **Pilates Seal** (see Video 16.3) as you invert your feet to bring the soles of your feet together. Like eversion, inversion is not typically a stable position; in fact, it makes one more susceptible to injury because it has a greater range of motion and also because the lateral ligaments do not stabilize the lateral aspect of the ankle as well as the deltoid ligament stabilizes the medial aspect (see Clinical Focus 15.1, Ankle Sprains).

Approximate Range of Motion

25 degrees

Muscles and Innervation

See Fig. 16.11.

Muscle	Nerve
Tibialis anterior	Deep fibular n. (L4, L5)
Tibialis posterior	Tibial n. (L4, L5)
Flexor digitorum longus	Tibial n. (S2, S3)
Flexor hallucis longus	Tibial n. (S2, S3)

Moving AnatoME Exercise
Foot Inversion: Pilates Seal

See Fig. 16.12 and Video 16.3.
- Starting position: Sitting on the floor in a "butterfly position" with hips externally rotated, knees flexed, and feet inverted so the soles of the feet contact one another. Engage your core as you flex your spine into a C-curve, rolling off of your sitting bones. Using your core, lift your feet off the ground, keeping the soles together. Bring your hands through the diamond shape made by your legs, and cradle the lateral aspects of your feet and ankles with your hands.
- Inhale to prepare.
- Without moving your spine, exhale in a staccato pattern for three beats as you abduct and adduct the hips, bringing the soles of the feet away from and toward the midline to touch on each exhale (as if you were a seal clapping its flippers).
- Inhale, and engage your core as you roll backward, maintaining the C-curve shape of your spine. Roll through your lumbar and thoracic spine until you come to balance on your upper thoracic spine (there should not be any pressure on your cervical spine).
- Balancing in this position, exhale in a staccato pattern for three beats as you abduct and adduct the hips, bringing the soles of the feet away from and toward the midline to touch on each exhale.
- Inhale, and rock back into the starting position.
- Repeat six to eight times.
- Ending position: Place your feet on the floor and return to a butterfly position.

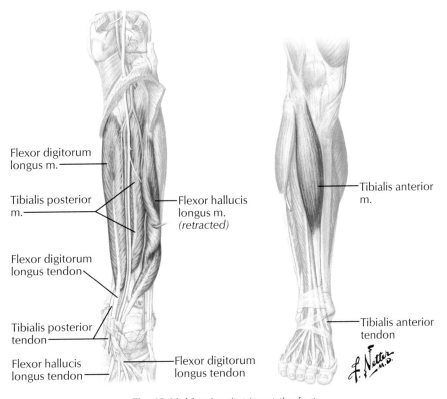

Flexor digitorum longus m.

Tibialis posterior m.

Flexor hallucis longus m. *(retracted)*

Flexor digitorum longus tendon

Tibialis posterior tendon

Flexor hallucis longus tendon

Flexor digitorum longus tendon

Tibialis anterior m.

Tibialis anterior tendon

Fig. 16.11 Muscles that invert the foot.

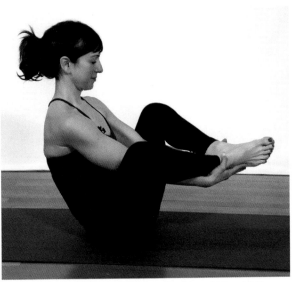

Fig. 16.12 Foot inversion: **Pilates Seal** (see Video 16.3).

17

Practical Applications of Moving AnatoME

As a student of health, your job is to understand the human body and learn about its structures and functions, requirements for good health, and deficits that may lead to poor health. This is important knowledge that you will use throughout your career on behalf of others and, we hope, yourself.

In an academic context, this knowledge is obtained from many sources, as you listen to lectures, read texts, and interface with patients. Additionally, your body is your own valuable learning tool; by experiencing its movements, you gain more understanding of information gleaned in the classroom. For example, performing a **Pilates Swimming** (see Video 13.3) gives you a physical memory of the location of the hip extensors in your body; it also gives you a lifelong "cheat sheet" that could help on a musculoskeletal exam one day.

There are intangible benefits derived from the integration of book and body, as well. One is increased body awareness; recognition of your own patterns and habits is crucial to maintaining health and preventing injury. Another benefit is personal accountability and the associated understanding of what a commitment to health requires; for instance, scheduling time in your calendar to go jogging, even if it means that you get less work done, and that you ask a friend to meet you so you are accountable for showing up. It can make the difference between knowing what you "should" do and actually doing it (eg, knowing that vegetables are good for you versus incorporating them into your diet). Practicing what you preach may also make you a more effective health practitioner. In fact, some studies have shown that sustaining your own healthy regimen helps you transmit lifestyle modification advice more effectively to your patient population.

Studies are also demonstrating the connections between a sound body and a sound mind. Some have shown that the body can provide a pathway to a greater sense of well-being. Following this pathway is especially important in the context of your studies; as a student of health today, the stress cards are stacked against you. As you take test after test, study and work for long hours, and sit up through sleepless nights, your academic pursuits take a toll. If you do not prioritize your own health, unhealthy habits can lead to conditions such as anxiety or lower back pain. However, they do not have to; you can reshuffle the cards you have been dealt by establishing self-care practices early in your academic and professional life. Just as there are streamlined tips on how to study for tests, there are also tried-and-true suggestions on how to practice self-care, a few of which are referenced in Chapter 18, Foundations for Health.

The onus is on you to take responsibility for your own health, as it is for each of your patients. When you not only learn about your body but also care for it, you both improve the quality of your life and tap into the incredible potential of leading by example. Nowhere in the Hippocratic Oath does it state "Do as I say, not as I do." So start small, begin with one health practice, and let your new pattern naturally expand. Over time, your understanding of *the* human body and *your* human body will grow together.

18

Foundations for Health: Posture and Mindfulness

There are many foundations for health. Two of them—posture and mindfulness—are effective and convenient within the course of your day.

POSTURE

You are living anatomy. Every muscle and bone you learned about in this book resides within you. Every second of every day, neurons fire, muscles contract, joints glide, and bones move, allowing you to interact with the world around you. Just as your body enables you to make a personal impact, it also receives a variety of impacts from each of your activities. So, as you learn about anatomy and its role in your patients' health care, what can you do to acknowledge your own anatomy and self-care?

When taking care of your body, having proper posture is a good place to start. A healthy posture promotes the proper alignment of the framework of *your* body. It also buttresses you from the repetitive stresses of your daily demands, whether from prolonged standing during rounds, writing notes, or moving clinical equipment.

What, exactly, is meant by *posture*? In 1947, The American Academy of Orthopedic Surgeons founded a Posture Committee, which defined posture as "the relative arrangement of the parts of the body." In her textbook *Muscle Testing and Function*, Florence Peterson Kendall, a pioneering physical therapist, further explained posture as "the composite of the positions of all the joints of the body at any given moment." Indeed, posture fits both of these definitions and others, as well. From an objective standpoint, we can easily observe the relationship of one joint to another and even classify different types of postures as (1) static (eg, standing in anatomical position), (2) dynamic (eg, the position when one is running), (3) an evolution in one position (eg, refining a yoga pose),

or (4) making a transition from one position to another (eg, rising from a sitting to a standing position). Subjectively, posture is harder to assess. Thinking about posture can be an ongoing lesson in personal physical awareness: Are my shoulders slouching? Is my pelvis tucked under me? Am I leaning into my right hip?

Posture not only varies by position, but also by activity, age, gender, genetics, culture, muscular condition, and other features. It is so uniquely and intimately associated with an individual at a particular point in time that no two postures are ever exactly the same.

Proper Posture

At the most general level, proper posture is that which promotes efficient alignment of your body at the cost of minimal energy expenditure, stress, and strain (Clinical Focus 18.1). This means, for example, that there is an ideal way for you to stand (and sit and run) that requires the least amount of your body's effort. Practice the following exercises to gain awareness of your postural habits and learn how to correct them as you move throughout your day (Box 18.1).

Moving AnatoME

Standing Posture: Yoga Mountain Pose (Tadasana) See Fig. 18.1 and Video 18.1.

An ideal standing posture is similar to anatomical position, with the exception of the placement of the feet and hands. In anatomical position, the feet are parallel to one another, toes pointing straight ahead; for most individuals, this position is more energetically costly than the foot position found in an ideal standing posture, with the feet approximating parallel and toes angled slightly outward. Also, in anatomical position, the palms of the hands are facing anteriorly; most individuals hold

CLINICAL FOCUS 18.1 Bad Posture

What happens when good posture does not? A musculoskeletal deviation resulting in physiologic inefficiency. Faulty alignment results in undue stress on the body's bones, joints, ligaments, and muscles. This stress not only impacts the improperly aligned region, but because our body is an interconnected whole, it negatively affects adjoining body parts, as well. Stress and strain from improper posture arise from the misuse of muscles, ligaments, and related structures; when firing inappropriately over long periods of time, some muscles elongate and weaken, whereas others shorten and tighten. Take, for example, excessive thoracic kyphosis, and the burden on the torso as the anterior thoracoappendicular muscles tighten and the posterior back extensors weaken (potentially compromising the respiratory organs, as well); this burden is also borne by the posterior neck extensors, which hyperextend the cervical spine so that one can maintain an eye level focus. Additionally, the lumbar spine counterbalances the thoracic flexion with excessive lordosis; as a result, the pelvis tips anteriorly, creating shortened hip flexors and elongated hip extensors. The biomechanical chain of strain continues on and on, until a simple slouch ends up as tendinitis of the hip.

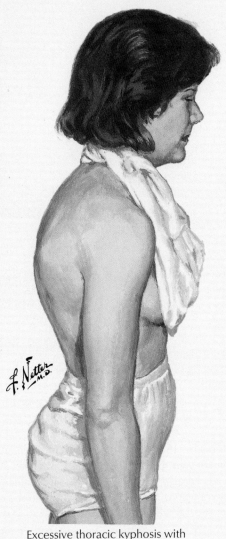

Excessive thoracic kyphosis with
compensatory lumbar lordosis

The ideal standing position may be best understood and standardized in reference to the line of gravity. The force of gravity travels down the standing body in an approximate line formed from the intersection of the sagittal and frontal planes in the midline of the body; around this line, the body is in a hypothetical state of equilibrium. A plumb line (a weighted cord) is used to represent this line of gravity. When one is viewing a patient anteriorly, posteriorly, or laterally, the line provides a standard for assessing the ideal standing alignment and measuring deviations from it. In ideal standing alignment, bony landmarks and anatomical points of reference of the patient (eg, the lateral malleolus) correspond to reference points on the plumb line. Faulty alignment occurs when the reference points deviate from the plumb line, increasing the risk for wear and tear on the body.

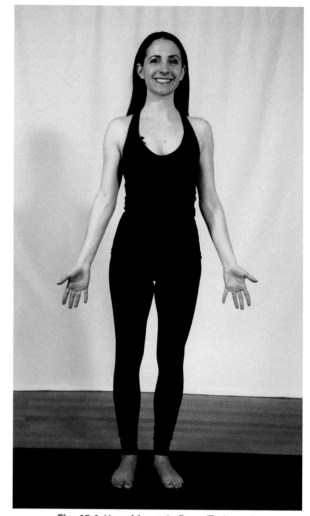

Fig. 18.1 Yoga Mountain Pose (Tadasana).

them in a more relaxed stance, facing medially. Practice your ideal standing posture with the **Yoga Mountain Pose (Tadasana)** (see Video 18.1). This core stance approximates anatomical position and is foundational for many yoga poses and sequences. It also provides awareness for you on how you stand, sit, bend, lift, and otherwise move through your day.

- Starting position: Standing with your feet hip distance apart, in their natural parallel position. Weight is centered between both feet. Arms relax by your sides.
- Form a firm foundation by spreading your toes on the floor. Engage the arches of both feet, and feel that engagement rise through your legs and thighs. Isometrically rotate your thighs inward.
- Lengthen your sitting bones toward the floor while elongating through the crown of your head.
- Engage your core so that it remains a center of strength.
- Gently open your chest and shoulders; feel your scapulae stabilized against your back. Forearms are engaged by your sides, with palms facing anteriorly and fingers extended.
- Align your neck on top of your torso, so that your cervical spine is a natural continuation of your thoracic spine. Your head rests in neutral, chin parallel to the floor. Release any neck and shoulder tension.
- Find one point of focus in front of you, soften your gaze, and breathe for five counts.
- Ending position: Exhale and return to your regular stance.

Sitting Posture: Computer Desk Station

See Fig. 18.2 and Video 18.2.

Sitting in front of a computer for long stretches is common in modern daily life. Learn how to do it properly and reduce the risk of chronic stress and strain.

- Place your chair 18 to 24 inches away from the computer screen.
- Place your feet flat on the floor, or on a footrest, in a natural parallel position.
- Position your knees directly over or slightly behind your ankles. Make sure that your knees are not flexed more than 90 degrees.
- Keep your thighs parallel, and position your hips so they are not flexed more than 90 degrees (you may

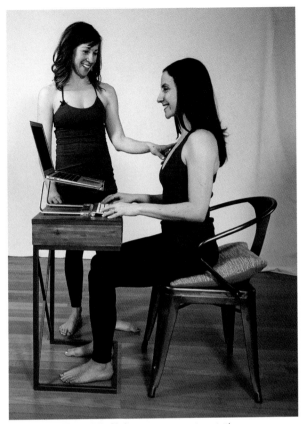

Fig. 18.2 Sitting at a computer station.

need to raise or lower your seat to achieve this). It is best to avoid crossing your legs; if you do cross them, alternate the leg on top to prevent imbalance.

- Sit directly and evenly on your sitting bones.
- Keep your torso erect, not leaning too far forward or back; maintain the lordotic curve of the lumbar spine with your pelvis in a neutral position.
- Maintain a neutral cervical spine; position the top of your computer screen so that it is at or slightly below eye level and you can keep your chin parallel to the ground (you may need to raise the height of the computer screen to accomplish this posture). Be aware of how positioning your eyes subtly positions your head and neck.
- Stack your shoulders over your hips. Broaden your chest and relax your shoulders, maintaining space between them and your ears.
- Flex your elbows to 90 degrees, so that your forearms are parallel to the floor.

- Place your wrists on the same plane as your elbows, in a neutral position, so they are neither flexed nor extended.
- Overall, maintain a posture that is active and engaged but not tense or gripped.

Use ergonomic supports, as necessary, to achieve proper positioning (eg, lumbar pads for sitting, wrist pads for typing). Remember that the body is not made to stay in one position for prolonged periods of time, no matter how proper the posture. Take postural breaks every 30 to 60 minutes by standing up or walking around. Likewise, take a 20-second vision break from your screen every 20 minutes by looking at an object 20 feet in the distance (20-20-20 rule). You can also shift positions while sitting, maintaining awareness of where your body is in space and which positions are most comfortable for you.

Dynamic Posture: Bending and Lifting

See Fig. 18.3 and Video 18.3.

Maximize your lifting power while minimizing bodily stress (eg, when lifting a patient onto a gurney) by practicing ideal bending and lifting posture.

- Respect your limits and lift only what you can safely handle.
- Before lifting, place your feet flat on the floor in a wide, firm stance close to the load. Gently bend your knees while maintaining an upright torso. Engage your core to protect your back. When possible, lift and carry at waist height. To bring the object to waist height, flex at the knees and the hips, maintaining a neutral and supported spine.
- Lift the load using lower extremity and gluteal strength to extend the hips and stand. You can then narrow your stance back to hip width (for walking, etc.), maintaining gently flexed knees.
- Keep your shoulders depressed, with your scapulae stabilized on your back.
- Hold the load close to your body. Flex at the elbows but keep your wrists neutral for maximum leverage and minimal damage.
- To lower the object, return to a wide, firm stance with flexed knees and neutral spine. Further flex the knees and hips to lower the object; do not flex through the spine.
- Return slowly to a standing position.

As a general rule of thumb, engage your core (see Chapter 6, Neck and Back) to protect your back. At all

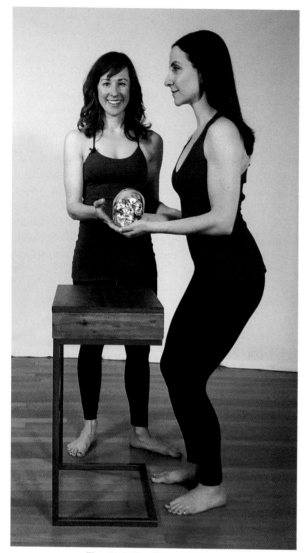

Fig. 18.3 Bending and lifting.

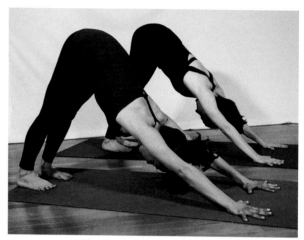

Fig. 18.4 Yoga and Pilates Flow.

costs, resist the temptation to flex from the vertebral column. Bending should occur primarily at the knee and hip joints, while you maintain a relatively neutral spine. Also, do not twist or rotate your torso while lifting and carrying a load. If you need to turn around, take small steps in the direction you need to go (Box 18.2).

Putting It All Together: Yoga and Pilates Flow

See Fig. 18.4 and Video 18.4.

How can you stand, sit, and lift properly when gravity is perpetually pulling you down? Ideally, ligaments alone should provide the support necessary to maintain proper

---

BOX 18.2 **Posture and Your Pelvis**

A key component of proper posture is the position of the pelvis, as it affects alignment of the lower limbs below and the torso and upper limbs above. An anatomically neutral pelvis, as defined by Florence Kendall, occurs when both anterior superior iliac spines lie in the same horizontal plane and the pubic symphysis and anterior superior iliac spines lie in the same vertical plane. Although some debate on the definition of a neutral pelvis exists, most professionals agree on the opposing muscles groups that exert balancing forces on the pelvis to effectuate proper posture throughout the rest of the body. These opposing muscles arise from the anterior and posterior trunk and thighs, both superiorly and inferiorly to the pelvis. For instance, the abdominal wall muscles (eg, rectus abdominis) flex the spine on the anterior pelvis to tilt it *posteriorly*, thereby extending the hips; the back muscles (eg, erector spinae), meanwhile, extend the spine, pulling on the posterior pelvis to tilt it *anteriorly*, thereby flexing the hips. Likewise, the hip joint flexors (eg, rectus femoris) pull on the anterior pelvis to tilt it *anteriorly*, thereby flexing the hips; and the hip joint extensors (eg, semitendinosus, gluteus maximus), conversely, pull *down* on the pelvis to tilt it *posteriorly*, thereby extending the hips. A neutral pelvis is often hard to achieve, as imbalances between these opposing muscle groups commonly occur due to poor posture during daily activities and/or poor conditioning. When striving for a neutral pelvis as part of proper posture, keep a balance of these muscles in mind.

posture, as ligamentous energy is less "expensive" than muscular energy and thus more physiologically efficient. In the real world, however, ideal circumstances are rarely present and individual idiosyncrasies almost always are; muscles, therefore, usually fire to maintain an upright posture, even when a person is in a passive stance. These muscles counteract the force of gravity and are therefore known by the nickname *antigravity muscles* (see Fig. 18.1). To enhance your posture, strengthen and stretch these muscles with the **Yoga and Pilates Flow,** which can be done as both a study tool and a study break.

- Starting position: Lying supine on the floor, with legs elongated and arms by your sides.
- **Pilates Pelvic Tilts** (see Video 13.2)
- **Pilates Roll-Up** (see Video 6.1)
- **Yoga Cat-Cow Pose (Marjaryasana-Bitilasana)** (see Video 8.2)
- **Pilates Leg Pull Prep** (see Video 10.2)
- **Yoga Downward-Facing Dog Pose (Adho Mukha Svanasana)** (see Video 11.2)
- **Yoga Plank Pose (Phalakasana)** (see Video 8.4)
- **Yoga Cobra Pose (Bhujangasana)** (see Video 6.2)
- **Pilates Swimming** (see Video 13.3)
- Ending position: Sit back into a resting pose with your knees and hips flexed, buttocks on your heels, and torso and arms elongated in front of you. Take a few deep breaths and then return to a comfortable cross-legged seat.

Use this sequence of poses as a foundation from which to customize your own flow. Feel free to repeat poses or to omit some poses and use others.

MINDFULNESS

Beyond physical demands, there is an emotional toll involved in patient care, as well. From the number of individuals you care for, to the number of individuals you work with on your team, plus all of the administrative responsibilities required, the stresses add up. It can be easy to feel distracted and overwhelmed.

Mindfulness can help you manage these feelings. By helping you to be present in the present, mindfulness helps you attune to and handle the stimuli of your environment (thoughts, emotions, sounds, sights, etc.) while centering yourself in it. In this way, your perceptions and behaviors focus on the present (versus the future or past) so you can respond appropriately and efficiently to the matter at hand.

> **PRACTICE WHAT YOU PREACH 18.1**
> **A Word to the Wise**
>
> There is no one way to become mindful. There are many methods available, and you may need to try a few to find what works for you (recognizing, as well, that what works for you now will change over time). Some easy ways to be mindful while you're at work include closing your eyes and taking five deep breaths, taking a quick walk around the block, standing barefoot on the grass somewhere close to your work, or scribbling your stream-of-consciousness thoughts in a journal at the start or end of your day. The important thing is to do *something* (even for 2 minutes), so start small with one technique and let the practice grow naturally from there.

The best way to understand mindfulness is through experience because it is highly subjective. Mindfulness can be a natural human attribute, and it can also be cultivated through specific techniques (Practice What You Preach 18.1). Focusing on your breath, for instance, is a popular technique. When encountering a stressful situation, have you ever been told to "just take a few deep breaths" before responding? Rather than just being unsolicited counsel, this sage advice has an actual physiologic basis. Slow, deep breathing stimulates on the parasympathetic division of your nervous system, or the "rest-and-digest response," which helps you feel calm and centered, which is a more optimal state to respond from. Like the development of any other skills, using your breath as a calming technique takes practice.

Meditation is likewise a popular mindfulness tool, as it serves to quiet the mind through disciplined concentration. There are many different forms, such as zen (zazen), transcendental, vipassana, mantra, and loving-kindness meditations. Researchers speculate that meditation may have originated with primitive hunter-gatherer peoples, who inadvertently discovered a meditative focus while staring at the flames of a fire.

Regardless of the mindful modality you choose, consistency is key, as it is with any pattern change. So be practical and patient, and remember that the most important part of any practice is showing up to do it. If a 1-minute meditation is your starting point, then start there. Over time, your practice will naturally lengthen, and 6 months from now you will have a new healthy habit to keep building from (versus continuing to wait until you can "find the time" to do it). Practice mindfulness with the following techniques that highlight breath, meditation, and movement.

Moving AnatoME

Deep Breathing Technique: Yoga Alternate Nostril Breath (Anuloma Viloma)

See Fig. 18.5 and Video 18.5.

- Starting position: Sitting in a comfortable cross-legged seat on the floor. If needed, support yourself with a cushion or on a chair. Set an alarm for 5 minutes and silence any other sounds (eg, phone ringer, computer).

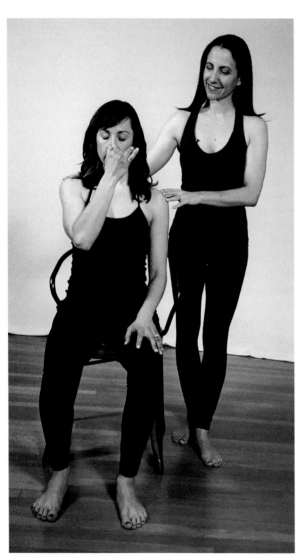

Fig. 18.5 Yoga Alternate Nostril Breath (Anuloma Viloma).

- Rest your left hand in your lap with the palm facing up. With your right hand, flex the index and middle fingers toward the palm while the thumb, ring, and pinky fingers extend.
- Close your eyes and take a couple of deep breaths through the nose.
- Following an exhale, gently close your right nostril with your right thumb; inhale through your left nostril for a slow count of four.
- Close your left nostril with your right ring finger.
- Retain your breath for a count of four.
- Open your right nostril and exhale slowly for four counts; modulate the exhale to last evenly throughout.
- Inhale for four counts through your right nostril.
- Close your right nostril with your right thumb.
- Retain your breath for a count of four.
- Open your left nostril and exhale slowly for four counts.
- Begin the cycle again, and repeat until the timer sounds.
- Ending position: Release your right hand onto your lap and return to your regular breath before arising.

Becoming Attuned to Your Environment:
Sensory Meditation

See Fig. 18.6 and Video 18.6.

Note that any of your five senses—sight, smell, touch, taste, hearing—can be used as the basis for this meditation. The following example uses sound to help your mind move from its machinations toward a central point of focus.

- Sit in a comfortable cross-legged seat on the floor or a chair (feel free to add cushions and supports, as necessary). The best seat is one that can healthily support you for the duration of the practice.
- Turn off your phone and set a timed alarm for 5, 10, or 20 minutes.
- Rest your hands in your lap, palms facing up. Gently close your eyes.
- Tune in to your environment and all the sounds therein.
- Focus your mind on one sound that is occurring around you (eg, outside traffic, chatter, beeping machine). Keep your attention on the sound by continuing to listen to it.
- When your mind wanders, catch it as soon as possible and bring it back to your chosen sound. Do not feel defeated if your mind wanders; most minds do. A sustained focus takes regular practice, which is why meditation is considered a practice.

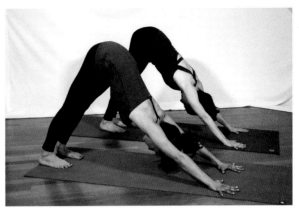
Fig. 18.7 Yoga and Pilates Flow.

- Remain seated until your alarm sounds. Pause for a moment to reflect on your experience before continuing with your day.

Putting It All Together: Yoga and Pilates Flow

See Fig. 18.7 and Video 18.4.

In yoga, focused concentration is called *dharana*. It is a practice in which you hone your thoughts by concentrating on a single mental object. Just like you attuned your awareness to the sense of sound in the prior meditation, you can also cultivate mindfulness by attuning to your own anatomy. Perform this sequence with a focus on whatever appeals to you at the time (eg, foot placement, your breath, a sense of calm); maintain the focus for the duration of this flow. If and when your mind wanders, bring it back to your chosen focus. In time, your ability to focus will increase both on the mat and throughout the rest of your day, as well.

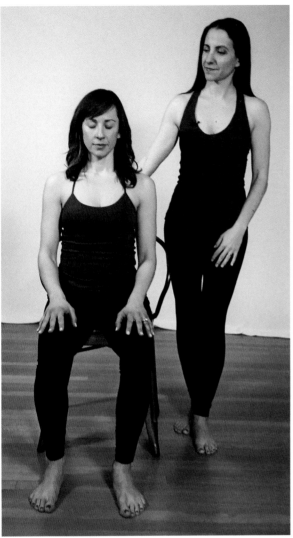
Fig. 18.6 Sensory meditation.

Clinical Focus and
Practice What You Preach Boxes

INDEX

Page numbers followed by "*f*" indicate figures, "*t*" indicate tables, and "*b*" indicate boxes.